W9-CCJ-193

# HEADACHES AREN'T FOREVER

by Dr. Gerald H. Smith

International Center for Nutritional Research, Inc.
40 Court Street
Newtown, PA 18940

Copyright© 1986 by Dr. Gerald H. Smith

All rights reserved. Permission to reproduce material from this book in any form must be obtained from the publisher. No part of this book may be reproduced in any form or by any means, electronic or mechnical, including photocopy, mimeographic or any information storage and retrieval system without the written permission of the publisher.

First printing, December 1986

Library of Congress Catalog Card Number: 86-83087
ISBN: 0-9617838-0-X

Published by International Center for Nutritional Research,Inc.
40 Court Street
Newtown, PA 18940

Edited by Gloria Brown
Cover designed by Patricia Pennington
Cover copy by Susan Soffer
Back cover copy by Blanche Schlessinger
Book composition by LD Graphics
Illustrations by Dr. Gerald H. Smith
Author's photograph by Britt Lewis Studios

# DEDICATION

It is a rare occurrence that our life's journey brings us in contact with an individual who has an altruistic mission. I consider myself blessed to have had the good fortune of many such personal interactions. Although many great minds have influenced my thinking, the one individual who has had the greatest impact on my professional career is Dr. Major B. DeJarnette. I extend tremendous gratitude to Dr. DeJarnette, the founder of one of chiropractic's more notable concepts, the Sacro Occipital Technic. Dedication of this book is my humble way of bestowing on this man the recognition he truly deserves.

While working for the Ford Motor Company as a young engineer, Dr. DeJarnette was severely injured by an explosion. The doctors gave him little chance of surviving, let alone recovering and being able to walk again. By the grace of God, Dr. DeJarnette was treated by the healing hands of an osteopath, William G. Sutherland. Miraculously, Dr. DeJarnette was healed through manipulation and upon his recovery made a lifelong commitment. This man went on to complete osteopathic training and then accepted the call to chiropractic. His inquisitiveness, genius, perseverance and unselfish desire to serve mankind led him to discover the reciprocal relationships of the skull bones, spine and pelvis to man's overall health.

Geniuses like Dr. DeJarnette are frequently rebuffed by their professional peers and establishment thinkers. He pressed on against all odds, even suffering the humiliation of being jailed as a result of actions by members of his own profession. The resentment, jealousy and fear of his accomplishments and great successes with hopeless patients followed him for much of his professional career. Dr. DeJarnette's untiring efforts, however, were not in vain. Throughout the world now, many chiropractors are performing his treatments and helping restore health to thousands of patients previously considered untreatable.

Dr. DeJarnette's work and his willingness to share his knowledge made this book possible. It is my firm conviction that one day this man's accomplishments will be recognized as monumental medical breakthroughs in the treatment of headaches and total body healing.

## Gerald H. Smith, B.S., D.D.S.
**author of** *Headaches Aren't Forever*

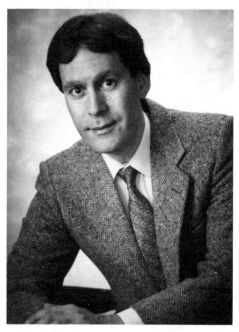

Gerald H. Smith is a recognized authority on craniomandibular somatic disorders–especially on pain therapy. Author of the landmark textbook for professionals, *Cranial-Dental-Sacral-Complex,* he now contributes an equally important guide for the lay person who needs to know how to cope with, control, and cure many kinds of headaches.

Doctor Smith's impressive list of credentals includes dozens of appearances as guest lecturer at national and international symposia, memberships in and affiliations with a number of professional associations such as the American Dental Association, International Association of Orthodontics, American Equilibration Society, Sacro-Occipital Research Society International . . . and many more. He was also past chairman of the Greater Delaware Valley Craniomandibular Research Study Group.

In addition, Smith is the originator of the CMA 1284™ (the world's first commercially available physiologic dental precision attachment that permits cranial bone motion) and originator of the concept of "dural fibrillation". And he's been awarded a U.S. patent for a flash adaptor to facilitate the taking of intra-oral photographs. Listed in *International Who's Who in Medicine,* Smith now shares his considerable expertise in this helpful book that is sure to bring blessed relief to thousands of headache sufferers.

**vii**

# TABLE OF CONTENTS
## Part I
### Understanding Basic Causes
### And Newer Methods Of Treating Headaches

## Part II
### Understanding The True Nature And
### Newer Methods Of Treating Migraine Headaches

## Part III
### A New Specialty Is Born

# Part IV
## Nutritional Aspects
## Of Headaches And Disease

# Part V
## Manipulation And Healing

# Part VI
## International Physician
## Referral Directory

# INTRODUCTION

Much has been written on the topic of headaches, their causes and cures. The concepts discussed in this book represent what the psychologist, Edward Debono, refers to as lateral thinking. Research energies were focused beyond the conventional causes and cures and resulted in a major discovery: The Physiologic Adaptive Range Concept. This concept integrates osteopathic, chiropractic, dental, physical therapy, and nutritional principles. It represents a major breakthrough in my twelve years of research and has generated new truths and culminated in a unique book that offers headache sufferers clinically proven, alternative, non-invasive therapies that bring relief in a high percentage of patients.

Truth goes through three stages before it is accepted. The first stage is **ridicule**. One of the most glaring examples in medical history involved an Austrian physician, Dr. Ignaz Semmelweiss. In the early 1840's, it was this physician's clinical observation that newborn infant mortalities were fewer within his own group of doctors and nurses than with other practitioners in the same hospital. Dr. Semmelweiss attributed his group's success to the fact that they washed their hands before going on to the next birthing patient. It was not the accepted medical wisdom at the time to wash one's hands between patients, and because he lacked double-blind studies Dr. Semmelweiss was rebuffed by his medical colleagues. He died in an insane asylum, a dejected and depressed man.

The second stage that truth must weather is **opposition.** Resistance at this phase stems from four factors. First, education establishes principles which the student must learn. These "truths" represent the efforts of establishment-oriented thinkers. In time, these principles become gospel and are used as yardsticks with which the student measures new information. Once entrenched, these principles become extremely difficult to change in textbooks. History reveals that a new idea will take at least fifty years before it is generally accepted as the "new gospel."

The second factor is ignorance. Sir William Osler, the great Canadian physician, summed it up when he stated, "The greater the ignorance the greater the dogmatism." Conventional thinkers usually offer the greatest resistance because of their myopic views. Thus, most health practitioners in search of a solution will keep digging a vertical hole within their own speciality. The innovative physician, however, has learned to dig laterally in other fields to find solutions to his patients' problems.

The third factor is insecurity. People do not like change and physicians are no exception. Learning and implementing new concepts in one's practice tend to upset one's *modus operandi.*

The final factor involves the extremely sensitive area of finances. Taking time off from practice, studying newer techniques and reducing the number of patients seen in a day cost dollars. The last thing any doctor wants is to have his rice bowl upset and his life style reduced.

The third stage that truth passes through is **self-evidence.** The excitement of employing a new concept is in watching it work. As more knowledge is gained, confidence grows and more people will be helped. This last stage can only occur if one is willing to take a chance and get involved.

When diagnostic tests have been exhausted, and the brain scans, magnetic resonance imaging, electroencephalographs, and allergy testing all come up negative, the headache sufferer must continue searching for relief. The following pages will provide fascinating insights into new sources and cures for acute and chronic headaches. Unfortunately, these areas have been overlooked by the majority of the medical and dental establishment, primarily because these concepts represent the new wave of emerging truths.

**Part I**

# Understanding Basic Causes
# And Newer Methods
# Of Treating Headaches

# PHYSIOLOGIC ADAPTIVE RANGE CONCEPT

The single most important function of the human body is maintaining a state of homeostasis or balance. The human body is constantly undergoing change both inside and out. In order to deal with the never-ending state of change, the body employs the brain which is the most sophisticated computer in the world. The receptors of the body act as the computer terminals and continually keep the brain informed of positional changes of limbs, blood pressure, temperature, acid-base balance of the blood, hormonal levels, mineral balance, toxic waste level, metabolism, and countless other processes.

The Physiologic Adaptive Range Concept is based on the premise that all structures (bones, ligaments, muscles, membranes, organs, nervous system, etc.), physiologic processes (digestion, blood formation, tissue repair, etc.), and fluids (enzymes, saliva, hormones, blood, urine, perspiration, etc.) function within an adaptable range. The body has the ability to compensate and maintain a state of balance within its genetic boundaries. Deviations beyond these physiologic adaptive ranges disrupt the body's homeostasis and shift function into a state of imbalance. If these imbalances persist, the body enters into a transition phase, which if not altered, progresses into a disease state.

To accomplish the incredible task of meeting all the demands, the body was architecturally designed to be self-correcting and contain all the machinery, chemicals, energy, healing and defense mechanisms necessary to maintain itself in excellent health.

As viewed by the Physiologic Adaptive Range Concept, the body functions with integration and biofeedback (hormonal and neurologic) mechanisms in five major areas:

1. Cranial Complex
2. Dental Complex
3. Pelvic Complex
4. Physiologic Complex (includes nervous system, muscle and ligament system, digestive system, lymphatic system, endocrine system, circulatory system, organs

of detoxification, reproductive system, etc.)
5. Psychologic Complex (includes mental well-being, capacity to cope with distress, and ability to be flexible under various circumstances)

Physiologically, the body functions within ranges in each of these major areas. Any textbook on physiology will contain specific laboratory values for these parameters:

1. Acid-base balance . . . . . . . . . . . . . .7.35 to 7.45
2. Blood calcium . . . . . . . . . .9.0 to 11.0 mg/100 ml
3. Cholesterol . . . . . . . . . . .150 to 250 mg/100 ml
4. Triglicerides . . . . . . . . . . . .0 to 150 mg/100 ml

Functionally, the body has ranges other than the blood values within which it maintains itself:

1. Body temperature: 96 degrees F to 99 degrees F
2. Blood pressure range for a 20 year old: 110/70-130/90
3. Cranial rhythm: 6 to 12 cycles per minute
4. Impulse firing of the central nervous system: 75 to 200 impulses per second
5. Muscle contraction time: 1/100 to 1/10 of a second (depending on the specific muscle)
6. Production of cerebrospinal fluid: 800 to 900 ml/ day
7. A muscle can stretch or contract within a 12 per cent range of its resting length.

There are many more areas that cannot be presently measured. In the near future, state of the art equipment sophistication will permit scientists to establish these ranges. Some examples are the vibratory rates of cells, auras of specific organs in health and disease, motion ranges of the dural membranes (surrounding the brain and spinal cord), and rate of energy flow along acupuncture meridians. These ranges will offer the physician of the future "normal" ranges similar to the blood studies that are presently available.

The internationally known chiropractic physician, Dr. George Goodheart, has a beautiful way of describing the function of the human body. Dr. Goodheart states, "The body is intricately simple and simply intricate." The body's ability to maintain the blood sugar level is a perfect case in point.

Blood sugar is maintained at a reasonably constant value of between 70 and 120 mg. per cent. This occurs despite the fact that irregular amounts of refined and complex carbohydrates (sugars), proteins, and fats are ingested at various times of the day.

Under normal circumstances, the adrenal glands, pancreas and liver function to produce hormones that work to control the blood sugar level. Ingestion of sugars raises the blood sugar level and signals the release of *insulin* which is produced by the pancreas (beta cells of the islets of Langerhans). Insulin lowers the blood sugar primarily by permitting the transport of glucose (blood sugar) through the cell membrane and into skeletal and heart muscle as well as fatty tissue. When the blood sugar level falls within the lower limits of the physiologic adaptive range, the body's balancing mechanisms activate.

Low sugar levels are also controlled by the pancreas (alpha cells), which produces a hormone, *glucagon.* In addition, the adrenal glands secret the hormone, *adrenalin,* which functions to slow down the action of insulin. Besides its inhibitive action, adrenalin causes a breakdown of stored liver and muscle starch which then produces the blood sugar, glucose. Of further significance, adrenalin stimulates the breakdown of triglycerides in fat tissue. The resulting fatty acids are then utilized by the cells thus sparing glucose supplies present in the blood plasma. Glucagon, although bearing no structural relationship to adrenalin, has a similar metabolic effect. Its release stimulates the breakdown of liver starch (glycogen), fatty tissue triglycerides, and formation of sugar (glucose) from amino acids. All these processes result in a blood sugar increase. As the blood sugar levels become elevated, the sugar acts directly on the pancreas to inhibit further release.

The fourth hormone factor is *cortisol* which is secreted by the adrenal gland. Cortisol increases the blood sugar level by inhibiting sugar uptake by many tissues. It also makes it easy for both muscle protein breakdown and conversion of the amino acids into sugar by the liver.

A delicate balance constantly exists within the body. As functions deviate within the physiologic ranges, the body remains in the relative state of health. When the body's adaptive ranges and self-correcting mechanisms are pushed beyond their capacity, physiologic chaos appears and the organism moves into a state of illness. The primary goal of the holistic physician is to remove as many structural, psychological and physiologic imbalances as quickly as possible to re-establish health. When the physician accomplishes this goal, the body is better able to function at its maximum potential and cope with the daily barrage of chemical, physical and psychological distresses.

## CRANIAL COMPLEX

The adult cranium contains twenty-eight bones: six middle ear bones, eight vault bones and fourteen facial bones. In the living state, these bones are constantly saturated with blood and exhibit a degree of flexibility. These cranial bones are joined together at junctions called sutures. These sutures are viable structures containing nerves, blood vessels, and fibrous connective tissue.

In the past, anatomists have viewed cranial sutures as immovable joints. This concept was developed after studying dried skulls and those of cadavers. It is a well known fact that at the time of death cranial motion ceases, sutures become restricted and the sutural ligaments calcify. However, the Drs. John Upledger, Ernest Retzlaff and Jon Vredevoogd, M.F.A. studied *living* skulls. (Diagnosis and Treatment of Temporoparietal Suture Head Pain: Journal of Osteopathic Medicine, July 1978, pp.19-26) These researchers conducted microscopic examinations of cranial suture material taken from living adults at the time of brain surgery. Their discovery of the viability of cranial sutures was established in the 1960s and presently is in the opposition stage of acceptance.

### THE ORTHODONTIC HEADACHE

Orthodontic treatment affects the cranium in 100 per cent of cases. Tooth movement and accompanying cranial bone changes may be beneficial, detrimental or may place stresses within the system without observable clinical symptoms. These latent structural imbalances will cause the body to be in a constant, active, adaptive state and often be the source

5

for chronic fatigue. In contrast, patients who are structurally balanced, that is, have a stable pelvis, spine, cranium and good tooth alignment will expend less energy to maintain body balance and overall are better able to cope with the stresses placed on their bodies.

Unfortunately, those patients whose body structure has been traumatized previously through the birthing process (forceps delivery, prolonged labor), physical trauma to the skull (fractures, blows, etc.), whiplash injuries, fractures of the pelvis, coccyx, legs, arms or other bones, traumatic dental extractions and surgical operations will have a greater likelihood for structural torquing or twisting of muscles, ligaments and other body parts. Structurally compensated orthodontic patients are the ones who will develop headaches soon after the braces and wires are placed. These head pains should not be confused with the temporary soreness and achiness that all patients will experience as a result of dental treatment. Patient complaints of chronic headaches, scalp tenderness, pains behind the eyes, muffled ear sounds, ringing, hissing or other ear distortions, balance problems, nausea, facial tightness, cervical or lower back pain or restriction of neck motion should all be thoroughly investigated for possible implication in cranial distortions, especially if they appear within days after braces are placed. Because of the body's tremendous capacity to adapt, these same symptoms may surface within a period of six months to several years.

## CASE STUDY

Astra came to my office in search of headache relief. She had been suffering head pains for the past seven years and had been existing on Excedrin. The 22-year-old student presented a list of medical diagnoses (from allergies to stress) offered at international pain clinics and by private practitioners. The patient told her doctors exactly what was wrong, however their lack of knowledge regarding the cranium caused them to dismiss the information as meaningless. Astra explicitly told her doctors that when she walked to school she would press her books on the top of her head to relieve her headache. In essence, the jammed cranial sutures were being released by the pressure of the books. A history of the patient's chief complaint revealed that orthodontic treatment had been instituted seven years earlier and that a night brace (headgear) had been used in treatment. Use of headgear has the potential effect of jamming cranial sutures. Relief came after two visits to my office. Gentle cranial manipulation was provided to release the jammed cranial sutures, which in turn have the effects of creating a torque in the dural membranes that surround the brain and disrupting cranial motion.

## ORTHODONTIC TIME BOMBS

### Case 1

JoAnne is a 44-year-old woman who came to my office seeking relief from chronic headaches which appeared immediately after a whiplash injury. The patient's dental examination revealed a malocclusion that had been previously treated orthodontically. The original dental problem involved a retruded lower jaw, a deep bite and horizontal protrusion of the upper front teeth. In dental terminology this represents a class II, division I malocclusion. Typically, these patients have an accompanying forward head posture and loss of the normal curvature of the cervical vertebrae. Conventional orthodontic therapy involved extracting the upper right and left first bicuspid teeth. This purely mechanical approach was aimed at achieving aesthetics only. In essence, the conventionally trained orthodontist amputated two teeth from a normal-sized upper jaw to make it correspond physically to a deficient lower jaw. The ensuing orthodontic treatment of moving back the upper six anterior teeth caused the restriction of the maxillae, palatine and sphenoid skull bones and created additional stress within an already tensioned dural tube. The physical trauma of the whiplash injury resulted in muscle spasms of the neck which would not respond to conventional drug or physical therapy. The patient's chronic headaches were being caused by the cervical dural torque which caused a reciprocal tension within the cranial dura. Treatment involved use of an orthopedic dental appliance which positioned the lower jaw downward and forward. This in turn helped restore the curvature of the cervical vertebrae, reduced the dural

7

tension and helped balance skull bone motion. JoAnne's chronic headaches were resolved and to date have not reappeared.

## Case 2

Tina is a 19-year-old college student whose chief complaints were that her jaw would periodically lock in a closed position, both jaw joints clicked during chewing and moderate to severe ear pains. These symptoms appeared immediately following trauma from an automobile accident. Clinical examination revealed that the patient had four first bicuspid teeth amputated to provide space in order to correct a dental malocclusion. Treatment at two university facial pain centers, plus numerous prescriptions for valium and muscle relaxers and an upper dental bite plate all failed to provide relief. The real problem, which had laid dormant until the accident, was caused by the conventional orthodontic treatment previously received. Mechanical tooth correction caused the lower jaw to be retruded and the bite to be overclosed. Tina's problems were corrected by bonding dental resins approximately one and one-half millimeters thick onto the biting surfaces of the posterior teeth. This increase of vertical tooth height helped establish a physiologic jaw position for the chewing muscles, provided space for the joint discs and reduced pressure on the nerves innervating the joint. Removing the causative factors resolved Tina's symptoms.

## Case 3

Renee was another victim of four first bicuspid amputation. As a young teenager, her malocclusion had been treated by conventional orthodontic wisdom. Removal of four teeth with retrusion of the lower jaw caused a distortion of her cervical vertebrae. Renee's body adapted well until age nineteen when two whiplash injuries within a year and a half upset the body's ability to adapt. Traumatic injuries from the second accident caused a tearing of tissue in the right temporomandibular joint. The resulting cervical muscle spasms caused the patient much difficulty in swallowing. For some time, Renee had been taking valium before eating to help her relax sufficiently to swallow her food. Chiropractic care, dental

8

support plus full body massage therapy were necessary to enable the patient to eat without the use of a drug. Because of irreversible soft tissue damage, surgery was performed and the right joint pain was eliminated.

## BIZARRE PATIENT BEHAVIOR

Periodically we hear reports of bizarre orthodontic patient behavior. These are the individuals who have forced orthodontists or general dentists to remove their braces at gun point. Locking one's cranium with orthodontic braces can be an extremely distressing physiologic experience. The individual's nervous system becomes overloaded with noxious impulses. This often results in feelings of severe agitation, anxiety, fatigue and exacerbation of low blood sugar symptoms of those afflicted. This abnormal behavior does in fact have a physiologic basis. Because cranial principles are not taught at the university level, most orthodontists, neurologists and other health professionals do not possess the knowledge needed to recognize the source of the problem and properly treat the patient. Even more appalling is the fact that many university-level professors deny the existence of cranial bone motion and the diverse effects of restricting bone movement.

## CRANIAL MOTION

Cranial motion was discovered in 1939 by an osteopath, William Sutherland. Research by Drs. Melicien Tettambel, David Michael and Ernest Retzlaff, Viola Fryman and others has substantiated the presence of cranial micro-motion. The origin of cranial motion is thought to be in the brain cells. The energy of contraction, relaxation, and expansion (cranial respiratory motion) takes place on a rhythmic basis just as with the lungs. Evidence indicates that there is a normal pulsile rhythm to all living cells. Our body is composed of 80 to 100 trillion cells, each capable of producing its own source of energy.

During cranial respiratory motion, the twenty-eight cranial bones function as a unit. The rhythmic micro-motion occurs within a physiologic range of six to twelve cycles per minute. This motion can be likened to an umbrella that is slowly opening and closing. The cranial motion itself is composed of two basic motions: primary and secondary. Primary motion involves the inherent movement of the brain and spinal cord, fluctuation of the cerebrospinal fluid, mobility of the intra-cranial and intra-spinal membranes, articular motion of the cranial bones and the involuntary mobility of the sacrum. Secondary cranial respiratory motion synchronizes with the body's breathing cycles of inhalation and exhalation. Inspiration causes a bilateral side-to-side expansion of the cranium, while expiration diminishes cranial size. This coordinated motion of primary and secondary respiration is accomplished by means of the dural membrane.

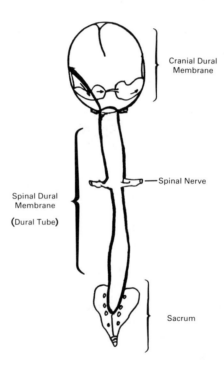

*Figure 1a.* The dural tube is a continuous membrane that surrounds the brain, passes out the base of the skull, attaches to the first three cervical vertebrae, and continues down the spinal cord where it finally attaches to the sacrum. This tube is the source for structural disturbances being transmitted from one part of the body to another. Because the body works reciprocally, imbalances in the skull can influence the neck, lower back, and pelvis and the reverse is also true.

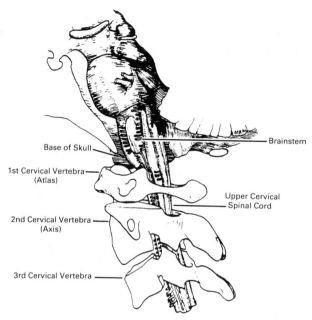

Base of Skull

Brainstem

1st Cervical Vertebra
(Atlas)

Upper Cervical
Spinal Cord

2nd Cervical Vertebra
(Axis)

3rd Cervical Vertebra

*Figure 1b. The upper cervical portion of the spinal cord and brainstem represent one of the most important areas of the nervous system. Within this area lie the automatic life sustaining centers—heartbeat, respiration, consciousness, and blood pressure. Also present are centers that control motor and sensory function to and from the face, eyes, mouth, and throat.*

*Distortion of the dural tube in this vital region has the potential to disrupt cerebrospinal fluid and blood flow to these important centers. Singly or in combination, the effects of vertebrae subluxations (malpositions), muscle spasms (due to tension or whiplash injury), dural tension from a rotated pelvis or a dental malocclusion will have far reaching motor and sensory disturbances throughout the body.*

If one visualizes the skull as a circus tent, then its supporting poles are the dural membranes. The dural membranes have a vertical and horizontal sickle-shaped component which allows reciprocal cranial bone motion between the sides and between front and back areas of the skull. Essentially, the cranial dura compartmentalizes the brain and furnishes it with a duct system (venous and cerebrospinal fluid) for irrigation, nourishment, and waste removal. Both cranial bone and dural membrane motion provide a synchronous pumping action that supports cerebrospinal fluid flow and insures the health of the entire body.

The dural membrane does not end within the cranium. It passes through the base of the skull, attaches to the first three cervical vertebrae and continues down the spinal cord and attaches to the sacrum (Fig. 1). The sacrum sits between two ilia and forms the pelvic complex. The significance of the sacrum is that it functions as a pump supplying pressure to insure flow of the cerebrospinal fluid up the central canal of the spinal cord back into the area of the brain.

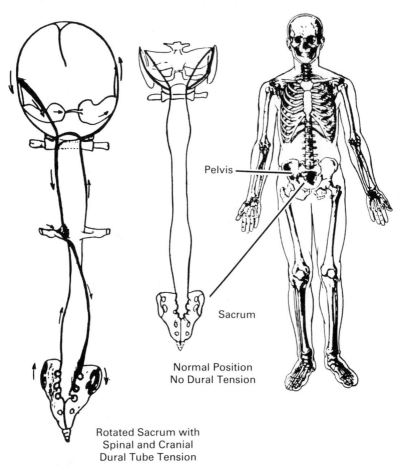

Pelvis

Sacrum

Normal Position
No Dural Tension

Rotated Sacrum with
Spinal and Cranial
Dural Tube Tension

*Figure 1c. In reality, the body functions just like a slinky. A distortion at one end will be reflected to its area of compensation. For example, the bones of the hands and feet work reciprocally as well as the ankle and wrist, knee and elbow, pelvis and shoulders. One of the main connecting links of the body that enables this slinky effect to occur is the dural tube. Joint receptors and neuromuscular biofeedback provide other means by which the body functions reciprocally.*

# Straws That Broke The Missionary's Back

## Case 1

Jane is a 49-year-old missionary who works in Alaska. Jane's accidental injury occurred in 1983 while helping a friend load bales of hay from a barn loft. An unexpected airborne bale struck Jane in the area of the right shoulder and neck. It wasn't until several months after the trauma that she suffered frequent neck and shoulder pain, shooting pains down the back of the spine and both arms, right hip pain, moderate pain over the right eye, decreased mobility of her neck, dizziness, chronic headaches and right arm weakness that prevented Jane from playing her accordion.

Chiropractic evaluation diagnosed Jane's symptoms as originating from muscle spasms, fascial irritation and a thoracic outlet syndrome. Manipulative care was successful in achieving a 40 per cent temporary improvement followed by a 10 to 15 per cent long term relief.

An orthopedic specialist was consulted after chiropractic care reached a healing plateau. Jane spent two weeks in the hospital where she underwent daily traction and physical therapy. An antidepressant with an anxiety-reducing, sedative component was given in the form of 100 mg. of Elavil at night. The drug was being used to help insure a deep, restful sleep. Additional temporary relief was achieved following the use of transthermal electrical stimulation to the neck and shoulder areas. Although some resolution of pain was achieved, Jane was still unable to regain full power back in her right arm.

A neurologist provided a third consultation and reaffirmed the diagnosis of a thoracic outlet syndrome. The prescribed continuation of physical therapy, however, was to no avail. Jane's symptoms persisted and it became obvious that a key factor was missing in treatment.

Jane was referred to a chiropractor in Spring House, Pennsylvania. Additional spinal and pelvic manipulation was instrumental in bringing more temporary relief. Again another

13

healing plateau was reached. The chiropractic physician referred Jane to a cardiologist who recommended further evaluation utilizing EMG, EKG, CAT scan, and magnetic resonance imaging (the latest in high technique soft and hard tissue imaging utilizing a strong magnetic field instead of conventional radiation). All the tests were negative. The chiropractor then referred Jane to my office for dental evaluation.

At the time of Jane's first visit to my office, she had been suffering with her original symptoms for the past three years. Presently, her only relief resulted from spinal manipulation followed by transcutaneous electrical nerve stimulation (TENS).

Dental examination revealed extensive cranial sutural jamming and an exceptional upper jaw (maxillae) width deficiency. This represented an orthopedic (bony) problem, rather than just crooked teeth, that pre-existed the 1983 traumatic injury. The narrow upper jaw was primarily the result of a genetic factor and from birth, Jane's upper cervical vertebrae, muscles, ligaments, remaining spine, pelvis and other associated structures adapted well to the existing structural imbalance. Nevertheless, the dural tube had a definite inherent strain, tension and torque. The injury to the right shoulder and neck upset the previous well-adapted structural balance. Because the scales were over-loaded on the side of imbalance, the body could not recover.

Treating Jane's structural imbalance required removing, as much as possible, the tension within the dural tube. This could only be accomplished by orthopedic expansion of the upper jaw by means of a dental orthopedic expansion appliance. While expansion was taking place, cranial manipulation was provided to release the jammed cranial sutures, soft laser acupuncture and myofascial release techniques were used to ease neck and shoulder muscle restrictions and nutritional therapy was provided to support tissue healing. Within three weeks after insertion of the appliance and adjunctive therapy, Jane started to regain strength in her right arm. The headaches were greatly reduced, the dizziness became much less frequent and she was now able to play the accordion for a minimum of a half hour. Because progress was significant, Jane returned home to Alaska where continuing dental and chiropractic care could be provided.

## "PSYCHOGENIC PARALYSIS"

### Case 2

Living under the influence of high levels of psychological distress coupled with structural imbalances will often lead to somatic disorders. This proved to be the Case with Stephanie. On the morning of June 7, 1986 Stephanie began to develop symptoms of pain and numbness in her left thigh. Several hours later, these symptoms involved the entire left leg, and the entire left upper extremity. It was under these conditions that Stephanie was rushed to the emergency room.

It was a day in June of 1986 that she will never forget. This once energetic 32-year-old university instructor was now lying in a hospital bed totally paralyzed on the left side of her body. The neurologist's report stated, " Motor examination revealed that the patient was unable to move the left arm or leg at all. She was unable to move even a finger, let alone lift the arm and leg off the bed. Sensory examination revealed markedly decreased appreciation of light touch and pinprick over the entire left arm, left side of the abdomen, thorax, left leg, and also the left side of the face." Stephanie became even more depressed when the CAT scan and electromyographic test results came back negative and the neurologist's diagnosis was left-sided paralysis of uncertain etiology.

Out of desperation, Stephanie's husband called me and requested a consultation. Since I was not on the hospital staff, I first had to obtain permission to examine the patient. After my examination, I concluded that Stephanie's paralysis was due to severe cervical, intra-oral and lumbar muscle spasms coupled with a sacroiliac distortion. My clinical experience has taught me that tensions such as these will affect the dural tube which in turn affect the cerebrospinal fluid and blood flow into the brain and spinal cord. Restriction of these vital fluids will cause neurologic motor and sensory deficits. For approximately one and one-half hours, I worked on relieving the cervical and intra-oral muscle spasms by employing gentle myofascial release techniques. During the last part of my therapy, I used cranial manipulation to restore the micro-motion back to the cranium. As I began releasing the various cranial restrictions, Stephanie began getting back the sensation in her left hand which was then followed by twitching in her index finger and thumb. At completion of therapy, Stephanie regained full strength, sensation and control of her left hand and arm. At this point, I recommended that her husband check Stephanie out of the hospital as soon as possible and seek the services of a competent chiropractor. Dramatic results were forthcoming following two chiropractic visits. After the second visit, Stephanie was able to drive and function like a normal person.

## Dural Fibrillation

It must be emphasized that all intra-cranial membranes are influenced by fascia (tough fibrous tissue that surrounds and covers all body parts), muscles, and skeletal stress. Changes at either the cranial or pelvic end, including spine distortions, will have a definite influence on the dural tube. The cranial dural sickles act as tent poles essential to the function of head movement and as stabilizers to the skull vault bones (Fig.2). These reciprocal tension membranes are themselves stabilized by the motion of the cranial base mechanism located at the junction of the occipital and sphenoid bones (sphenobasilar mechanism) which also balances the spinal membranes and provides a major pumping action for the cerebrospinal fluid. Dr. DeJarnette has described the reciprocal tension membranes of the spinal column and cranium as the balancing mechanism that permits coordination of the bony parts of each side of the skull and with the spinal vertebrae.

An imbalance of the cranial rhythm (dural fibrillation) will prove very distressing to the patient and even may prove totally disabling. Clinical symptoms may be exhibited in the form of mental confusion, stuttering, chronic headaches, disequilibrium, irrational fears, disruption of sleep pattern, fatigue, forgetfulness, hand tremors, agitation, sutural pain, cranial and facial tightness, scalp tenderness, eye motor dysfunction, color and visual perceptual distortions and many other neurological symptoms.

This author has come to realize the clinical significance of a dysfunctioning cranial dural membrane motion. Often overlooked is the patient whose chief complaints are lack of concentration, balance problems and facial and headache pain

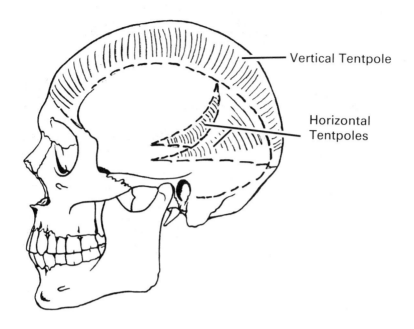

Vertical Tentpole

Horizontal
Tentpoles

*Figure 2. The cranial dural membranes act as stabilizers to the vault bones. Physical trauma (whiplash injuries, falls, blows to the head, forceful tooth extraction, etc.) and dental malocclusions have the potential to disrupt dural membrane balance and normal cranial rhythm. Such changes can cause adverse neurological function throughout the body.*

attributed to dural fibrillation. An irregular dural membrane motion can be the result of a whiplash injury, physical trauma to the cranium, spine or pelvis, a restricted cranium due to upper dental appliances (splinted upper fixed bridgework that crosses the mid-line or an upper cast partial denture) and traumatic or forceful tooth extraction. Such rhythm imbalances have the potential of placing pressure on cranial nerves and disrupting cerebrospinal fluid flow (thus impeding removal of metabolic wastes, flow of blood and nutrients, hormones, neurotransmitters, and other vital substances into and out of brain cells). Ultimately, cranial and sacral bone motion will be disrupted and accompanied by neurological, neuromuscular and organ symptomatology. When studying cranial dural anatomy, one realizes the full impact of the potential for disrupting central nervous system function.

# CASE 1

Susan is a 39-year-old school teacher who was involved in a motor vehicle accident. A whiplash injury occurred and was accompanied by facial pain, chronic post-occipital headaches, lack of concentration, irritability and chronic fatigue. The patient had been suffering these symptoms for a period of six weeks after her accident. A clinical examination revealed cranial bone distortions primarily on the right side, the cranial dura was in a state of fibrillation, and there was a distortion of the sacroiliac joint. Treatment involved gentle cranial manipulation which released sutural restrictions (juncture between skull bones) and balanced the cranial rhythm and dural membrane motion. Upon completion of therapy on the first visit, Susan's facial pains, post-occipital headaches and lack of mental acuity were immediately resolved.

# CASE 2

Mary, a 48-year-old executive secretary had committed herself to a 30-day program for alcohol detoxification and recuperation from occupational burnout. Mary's primary symptoms were depression, loss of mental acuity, loss of visual image sharpness, chronic fatigue (sleeping 12 to 14 hours a day without sedatives), upper cervical pains, disequilibrium, digestion problems, distorted and muffled auditory sounds, inability to function normally, lack of incentive, poor self image and lack of internal motivation.

Examination of the patient's cranium revealed extensive sutural jamming and a state of dural fibrillation. Dentally, the patient's upper jaw (maxillae) was restricted in its normal physiologic range of motion because of an upper fixed anterior bridge. A deep overbite (collapsed vertical), due to lack of posterior support of the teeth, further served as a complicating structural problem. The upper cervical vertebrae exhibited lack of normal mobility ranges accompanied by contracture and muscle spasms of the surrounding tissues. In addition, problems with the lower lumbar vertebrae and a weakness of the sacroiliac joint existed.

Treatment focused on correcting the cranial bone distortions, releasing the jammed cranial sutures, balancing the cranial rhythm and dural membrane motion, releasing the neck tightness using myofascial techniques, and providing proper dental support. The macrobiotic diet for detoxification and overall health was recommended to the patient.

Immediate success resulted from cranial manipulation therapy. The symptoms of a lack of mental acuity, disequilibrium and visual and auditory perceptual problems disappeared the next day. That night the patient slept soundly without drugs and awoke at 7:30 A.M. with mental acuity and no feelings of depression.

## CASE 3

One year and seven months prior to seeing Ruth she had been suffering from a list of seemingly bizarre symptoms. The 51-year-old patient was leaving the ladies room of a movie theatre when the heavy metal door struck her on the left side of the head. The trauma caused her to see orange stars and she became dazed for a moment after the incident. The force was sufficient enough to rip her left earring through the ear lobe. Her right eye began tearing so excessively that she had to remove the contact lens. The patient's left temporal area swelled and she slept poorly that night.

Following the accident, the patient continued to work for a few months. However, during that period, her symptoms became so severe that she had to terminate employment. Prior to cranial therapy the consulting neurologist recorded the following residual problems:

1. Stuttering
2. Difficulty coordinating thoughts
3. Depression and tension
4. Tremors of the hand
5. Impaired memory (The patient may forget what she was saying in the middle of a sentence. She may forget what she was looking for when she goes into her pocketbook. She forgets the names of people she knows.)
6. Impaired concentration

19

7. Pains in her jaws and ear canals
8. Pain in the back of the head above the ears
9. Vertex pain on the top of her head
10. Aching pain in the lower back region
11. Extreme fatigue
12. Difficulty staying asleep during the night
13. Abdominal pain
14. Blurred vision
15. Bright lights bother her
16. She has noise in her ears, "like the ocean."
17. Bad dreams at night
18. Appetite is poor
19. Some hair loss since the head injury

Clinical examination revealed the patient had extensive cranial bone distortions, jammed cranial sutures, an asynchronous cranial rhythm, dural fibrillation, a major dental problem in the form of a collapsed bite (due to absence of many posterior teeth), and a chronic sacroiliac weakness involving overstretching of the supporting ligaments. Prior to the accident the patient's body was in a constant active state of adaptation. Ruth's cranium was the principal area of compensation for all her structural defects. The physical trauma to the head took away her body's major compensatory mechanism for survival, and Ruth's system went into chaos. With a clinical history as presented, it is no wonder she was viewed as a hypochondriac and malingerer.

Treatment had the supreme objective of restoring the patient's compensatory mechanism – a cranium capable of functioning within a physiologic adaptive range. Osteopathic myofascial release techniques, which employ gentle tractioning of the cervical tissue, were used to relax the neck muscles. The patient's cranial primary and secondary respiratory rhythms were restored to physiologic harmony. Sacral occipital cranial techniques developed by Dr. DeJarnette were performed to correct cranial bone and sutural distortions. The released muscles permitted the cranial bones to properly function which then allowed the sutural system to respond, thus enabling the dural membranes to ease tensions which, when all totaled, established a more normal cerebrospinal fluid flow and neurologic function. The patient had dramatic results immediately following the first cranial manipulation. After the eighth cranial adjustment, the patient was free of most of her original post-trauma complaints.

A medical doctor who was board-certified in neurology and psychiatry re-examined the patient following cranial manipulation. When questioned about her original symptoms, the patient stated that she had immediate relief of many of her problems and she was able to discontinue taking the prescribed Elavil (a drug designed to modify states of depression). The neurologist reviewed Ruth's original symptoms and noted the following improvements:

1. There is no longer any stuttering.
2. She has less difficulty coordinating her thoughts.
3. She is not depressed and is less tense.
4. There is much less tremor.
5. The patient is less forgetful.
6. She has less difficulty concentrating.
7. There is diminished pain in the ears and in her jaws.
8. She has less pain in the back of her head and she is able to walk normally.
9. There is less frequent pain at the top of her head.
10. She seldom has pain in the lower back area.
11. She no longer feels as tired. Fatigue episodes have occurred only twice in the past ten days.
12. She now sleeps seven to eight hours normally.
13. There is much less abdominal pain.
14. She has no blurring of vision except when she tries to read.
15. There is less trouble with bright lights.
16. She very seldom hears noises in her ears.
17. She no longer is having bad dreams.
18. Her appetite is back to normal.
19. Her hair is no longer falling out and it is growing more rapidly.

Reviewing this patient's past medical history revealed an interesting piece of information. In 1976 Ruth was involved in an automobile accident and sustained head injuries. She had amnesia for the event, and suffered with severe headaches and experienced trouble with mental clarity for a three-year period. It is my opinion and clinical experience that symptoms of post-concussion syndrome are the consequences of disruption of cranial rhythm which results from the trauma. As the cerebrospinal fluid flow becomes disrupted, the potential for numerous neurological problems materializes. This patient's suffering could have been easily resolved if emergency room personnel had been capable of administering basic cranial therapy. Too often, post-whiplash patients are dismissed from the hospital with a prescription for Valium and a soft collar.

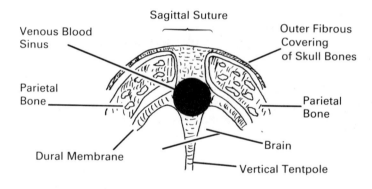

*Figure 3. Scientists have documented the existence of nerves, blood vessels and connecting fibers in the sutural areas. Anatomists have also shown the direct physical connection between the inside and outside of the skull. The dural membrane that surrounds the brain communicates with and influences the outside of the skull by means of an outer fibrous layer. This layer passes through the sutures and covers the bony portions of the skull. For this reason, internal tensions have the potential to cause external changes such as muscle spasms (sore scalp) and vice-type pressure. The reverse is also true. Whether the headache is due to physical tension or a vascular migraine, the dural membranes will be affected.*

Possessing even a superficial understanding of cranial anatomy and function as presented, one begins to appreciate the complexity of the human brain and its dysfunction with structural imbalances. Although not voluminous, scientific documentation regarding cranial micro-motion, cerebrospinal fluid flow, and sutural anatomy does appear in the professional literature. In the early 1960s sutural areas between cranial bones were documented by histologic methods to reveal blood vessels, nerve plexus surrounding the blood vessels, connective tissues, connecting fibers from soft tissue into the adjoining bone, and free nerve endings. Gross anatomic dissection by Dr. Marc Pick (SOT chiropractic physician, anatomist, international lecturer) clearly demonstrated that the outer layer of dural membrane that surrounds the brain passes through the suture and forms the fibrous outer layer (periosteum) which surrounds the skull bones. This architectural design permits coordination of cranial bone movement and internal tensions on the dural tentpoles (falx cerebelli, falx cerebri, and tentorium cerebelli). In the well-respected textbook, *Gray's Anatomy,* it is stated that these dural membranes are innervated by cranial and cervical nerves. This further substantiates the extensive biofeedback mechanism which constantly functions to maintain body balance. As various physical tensions develop, nervous impulses relay the information to the brain which then fires impulses to corresponding motor nerves which control the skeletal muscles effecting structural corrections.

## CRANIAL INVOLVEMENT IN NEWBORNS

An osteopathic physician, Viola Fryman, conducted a study on 1250 newborn infants. (Relation of Disturbances of Craniosacral Mechanisms to Symptomatology of the Newborn: Journal of American Osteopathic Association, 65:1059-1075, 1966.) Dr. Fryman, whose specialty focuses on dysfunctions of the cranium, observed that 10 per cent of the newborns had severe visible trauma inflicted on their heads while in utero or during labor. Cranial examination of the remaining infants revealed cranial bone strains in 78 per cent of the cases. The study concluded that nearly 90 per cent of all infants had cranial distortions that resulted while they were being carried or that occurred during delivery. Many of these babies were observed in the nursery to have problems with the sucking reflex, vomiting, nervous tension, irregular sleeping patterns, and irregular vital signs such as heart rate and breathing. Osteopathic and chiropractic physicians trained in cranial techniques can effectively treat many cranial bone distortions when infants are only three days old. If allowed to go untreated, these distortions have the potential of providing structural imbalances that can be the source of chronic headaches, hormonal imbalances and other neurological problems that occur during adolescence or adulthood.

## DURAL TORQUE HEADACHES

Carmen was referred to my office by her ear, nose and throat specialist. The 33-year-old school teacher had been suffering with facial and stabbing left ear pains. Her facial pain radiated across the entire left side of her face and was not responding to either the Antivert (drug given to alleviate balance problems) or anti-inflammatory medications. Although the symptoms had appeared two weeks prior to her visit, the patient was very distressed. My examination revealed that the patient's pelvis was rotated creating a functional short left leg. This in turn created in her sacrum a torque which was transmitted up the spinal dura (dural tube) into the skull. This ultimately caused the cranial bones and sutures on the left side to be jammed. If one visualizes the dural tube, which connects the pelvis and cranium, as a towel that becomes twisted and shortened, then one can easily understand how the face becomes affected on one side. All cranial nerves pass through the cranial dura. If the dura is under tension or torqued, then the nerves passing through will be affected and neurologic symtoms will appear. The patient's problem was aggravated by the fact that she slept on a double pillow. This caused her head to be thrust forward placing additional tension on the dural tube and accentuating the facial pain. Treatment consisted of balancing the patient's pelvis by means of padded wedges (part of the Sacro Occipital Technic established by Dr. De Jarnette) and releasing the cranial restrictions by gentle manipulation. The facial and ear pains disappeared during the first visit as soon as the pelvis and cranial sutures were balanced and dural tension released. The patient has not had a recurrence for over 18 months.

A torque or twisting type tension somewhere along the dural tube has the potential of pulling the cranial bones inward and jamming the sutural areas between the bones. This may result from a distortion of any of the spinal vertebrae, rotation of the pelvis or displacement of the coccyx (tail) bone due to fracture or trauma from a fall. Another source for jamming cranial sutures comes from the fascia. Fascia is connective tissue, composed primarily of collagenous and elastic fibers, which surrounds all muscles and other parts of the body. This fascia exists in a state of dynamic equilibrium as it surrounds the entire body. In reality, when the body becomes distorted from a whiplash injury, surgical- or trauma-induced scars, physical trauma or muscle tension, the fascia pulls tight around the body in much the same way that a cellophane wrapper responds to heat. As body muscula- ture tightens, especially the muscles of the upper shoulder and neck (muscle tension headache), the reactive muscles and fascia surrounding the cranium will compress the sutural areas. Because the sutural areas are composed of viable tissue, the outside surrounding fascia of the skull passes through the viable suture and becomes continuous with the dural membranes that surround the brain. The anatomical connection between internal and external structures becomes obvious. The significance of the muscle tension headache is derived from several key factors:

1. Muscles that are attached to cranial bones and are in spasm will put a drag on the normal cranial bone motion.

2. Spastic muscles that span cranial sutural areas will cause physical jamming.

3. A jammed sutural area will exhibit tissue anoxia (lack of oxygen) and will impinge on free nerve endings

25

(send pain signals) within the suture to cause localized pain.

4. Sutural jamming has the potential of creating tension
   in the dural membrane system thus affecting the flow
   of cerebrospinal fluid and blood.

5. Dural membrane tension has the potential of stimulating cranial nerves (parasympathetic nervous system)
   thus increasing production of histamine (causes dilation of blood vessels), cerebrospinal fluid and causing
   the throbbing pressure type headache.

## FASCIAL HEADACHE

Virginia is a 41-year-old housewife who was involved in an
automobile accident and as a result had been suffering for two
and a half years. The post-whiplash injuries caused chronic
headaches, neck pains, left shoulder pain, and right knee
pain. Severe muscle spasms of neck and shoulders prevented
the patient from fully rotating her head to the left and
resulted in bilateral sidebending restrictions.

Whiplash injuries to the spine may cause a hyperflexion
(extreme forward bending) and extension (backward) type of
lesion. In addition, a corkscrew effect may occur in the lower
lumbar vertebrae which also affects the sacroiliac joint. These
forward, backward, and twisting distortions set up muscle
spasm patterns that perpetuate bony structural and fascial
strains. Conventional healing methods use drugs, hot and
cold packs, and electrical stimulation which only serve to
mask the patient's symptoms.

Virginia's treatment focused on resolving the structural
imbalances of the sacroiliac, spastic muscles, and restricted
fascial sheaths. Myofascial release techniques were first used
to free up the patient's neck and shoulder tightness. As the
gentle manipulations released the cervical restrictions, the
spine and muscles began to assume a more normal posture.
Releasing the tissue tightness allowed the internal and
external fascial connections of the cranium to relax. After
Virginia's first treatment, the headaches were relieved. To
insure elimination of the muscle spasm problem, a regimen of

natural B-complex vitamins, unsaturated fatty acids and multi-minerals was taken. The patient was then referred for chiropractic care. Stability of the sacroiliac was achieved thus releasing tensions in the dural tube. Successful treatment using non-invasive techniques has enabled this patient to assume a normal life.

## CEREBROSPINAL FLUID

The cerebrospinal fluid (CSF), its production function, and flow represents a separate circulatory system in the body. Cerebrospinal fluid is not just a simple fluid designed to protect our brain. It represents one of the most complex fluids in our body. Scientists have discovered that CSF contains every bioactive substance known-- hormones, gland stimulating factors, nutrients, and nerve messengers. Scientific journals contain descriptions of numerous experiments pertaining to cerebrospinal fluid, but the general conclusion drawn is that CSF functions primarily to integrate messages and maintain a physiologic balance for the brain, spinal cord and peripheral nerves to sustain life.

Cerebrospinal fluid is produced by the choroid plexus that line the ventricles of the brain. Within a 24-hour period, approximately 800 to 900 ml. of CSF is produced. The measured volume of CSF that surrounds the brain and spinal cord is only 150 ml. These statistics substantiate the fact that CSF changes five to six times per day. As the brain expands synchronously with each inspiration of the lungs, CSF is released from the fourth ventricle of the brain. The fluid flows up around the brain hemispheres, down the spinal cord and out along each spinal nerve. Recent documentation by Dr. Marshal Rennels at the University of of Maryland has shown that the CSF is actually pumped into the brain tissue under pressure. The fluid takes four to five minutes to diffuse through the brain. In additional research, Steer and Horny have traced CSF using radioactive isotopes flowing into the organs and other structures that the nerve innervates. Of further interest is the fact that stimulation of the cranial nerves (parasympathetic portion of the nervous system) will cause an increase in the production of cerebrospinal fluid.

# CEREBROSPINAL FLUID PRESSURE HEADACHE

Carol was referred by her son-in-law, a general dentist. When I first examined the patient, Carol's endocrinologist had recommended that a tube be placed in her brain to drain excess CSF. Carol's problem stemmed from post-operative sequelae that resulted after the successful removal of a pituitary tumor. The neurosurgeon who performed the operation was reluctant to insert the shunt into the ventricle of the brain and strongly recommended seeking a conservative alternative. Intermittent headaches and limited jaw opening appeared immediately after surgery. Approximately three years following the initial surgery the patient developed constant headaches which she suffered for a year and a half. These head pains came in the form of a pressure build up within the skull accompanied by bilateral pain in the temporal area. The chronicity of the cranial pressure, pains, and limited mouth opening created a very distressful existence.

The practitioner who understands basic functional cranial anatomy and relates it to the trauma incurred during the operation will have insight into achieving a solution. The fact that the patient had been in the operating room for eight hours with her mouth propped open caused severe spasms of the jaw-opening muscles. These chewing muscles attach directly to cranial bones and when in spasm they restrict the normal cranial physiologic motion.

Treatment involved first relieving the muscle spasm problems then correcting the irregular cranial motion. Soft laser acupuncture was used to assist in the release of the associated muscle spasms. This painless, non-invasive technique employs an extremely low wattage laser energy source (1 milliwatt) coupled with a nonperceptible galvanic stimulation. This form of electromedicine is directed to the associated acupuncture and muscle trigger points. Myofascial release techniques were then used to reduce the existing cervical tissue tightness. Once the surrounding muscle and fascial restrictions were eased, direct attention was focused on the specific cranial bone distortions. Special emphasis was placed on establishing harmony of the cranial rhythm. This rhythm is essential for the cerebrospinal fluid to properly flow around and into all parts of the brain tissue for proper nourishment, waste removal, hormonal transfer and neurologic function. Balancing cranial rhythm and releasing sutural restrictions reduced stimulation of the parasympathetic nervous system (cranial nerves) which in turn established a more normal production of cerebrospinal fluid and eliminated the constant cranial pressure. After just one treatment session, Carol was able to open her mouth wide enough to bite into a large sandwich. The bilateral head pains disappeared immediately and within a week following initial cranial therapy the head pressure pains were completely gone. For adjunctive and maintenance treatment, Carol sought the services of an SOT (Sacro Occipital Technic) chiropractor.

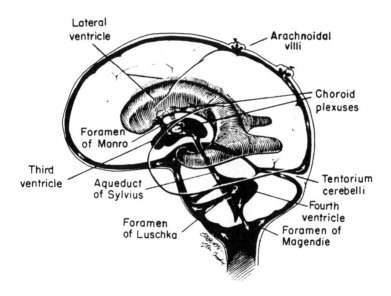

*Figure 4.* The cerebrospinal fluid (CSF) is produced by the choroid plexuses within the ventricles of the brain. Increased production occurs with increased stimulation of the parasympathetic (PNS) part of the nervous system. The PNS is located primarily in the cranium and sacral parts of the body. Distortions of the skull bones or pelvic area have the potential to cause an increased quantity of CSF and raise intracranial pressure.

Although discovered over fifty years ago, acceptance of the principles and practical applications of cranial manipulation has been slow in coming. As a non-invasive therapeutic approach, cranial techniques have resolved many medical problems which are presently being treated purely with drugs to mask the symptoms. Such maladies as migraine headaches, post-concussion syndrome, facial palsy, Bell's palsy, trigeminal neuralgia, tic douloureux, vertigo, tinnitis, seasickness, chronic earaches without infection, eye pain, jaw pain, sciatica, and idiopathic hypertension all have been lessened or totally resolved when structural cranial distortions are the cause.

# Part II

# Understanding The True Nature
# And Newer Methods
# Of Treating Migraine Headaches

# MIGRAINE HEADACHES

It has been estimated that approximately 25 million people suffer from migraine headaches. Its victims are all ages and are from all walks of life. Some of the more notable sufferers were the noted psychiatrist Sigmund Freud, novelist Lewis Carroll, philosopher Immanuel Kant and Paul, the Apostle.

The word "migraine" originated more than 2500 years ago during the time of Hippocrates. It was the Greek physician Galen in the second century A.D. who first called the malady "hemikrania," a Greek word meaning "half skull." The present day term migraine, was derived from the French. Commonly, the migraine headache is visualized as a throbbing, recurrent pain which affects one side of the head. Although the symptoms of migraine are varied, approximately 10 per cent of the victims suffer the more common classic form. Approximately two hours prior to the onset of pain, the patient experiences prodromal visual phenomena. These may consist of flashing or shimmering lights, visual floaters, zigzag patterns of lines, blind spots in the visual field, and even temporary loss of vision in one eye. Additional early signs may include paresthesia or tingling in an arm or foot that progressively spreads through a portion or entire half of the body on the opposite side where the migraine will strike. Accompanying these early warning signs, may be depression, feelings of helplessness, irritability and impending doom.

A two-hour period will usually pass after the initial symptoms and the beginning pain. The most frequent pain sites appear in the temporal areas, around one eye, or the forehead. Although migraine pain is usually limited to one side of the head, the sufferer may experience a switching of the pain to the opposite side during the same migraine attack or it may appear on the opposite side at a later attack.

Once started, the migraine pain progresses to a pulsating, pounding intolerable state. Duration of an untreated classical migraine ranges between four and six hours. As pain escalates and reaches its maximum level within two hours, the severity of the symptoms increases in direct proportion: extreme sensitivity occurs to bright lights and sounds, speech may become slurred, nausea and vomiting may develop, absence of appetite, loss of complexion and profuse sweating may predominate. The visual distortions and accompanying neurological dysfunctions have been attributed to decreased blood supply to the cerebral cortex region of the brain. The cerebral cortex lies near the brain surface and contains nerve cells that are responsible for vision, smell and auditory perception, writing, biological intelligence, body motor and sensory function.

Migraines are unique vascularly in that the larger arteries and veins dilate while the smaller vessels that carry the blood from the arteries to the veins constrict. This physiologic response follows a universal principle – for every action there is an equal and opposite reaction. The relative increase in blood flow occurs when the normal influx of blood into the head remains the same but the volume exiting diminishes. As the blood backs up within the skull, the larger arteries and veins become engorged. The decreased blood flow leaving the head is the result of muscle spasms at the base of the cranium. This reciprocal action is the body's means of maintaining balance. The greater the dilation the greater the reciprocal constriction must be of the smaller blood vessels. Although there is plenty of blood available in the brain, the quantity reaching the tissue at any one time is less than normal. This scenario accounts for the pounding head pain and various neurologic symptoms. Without such mechanisms, the body would remain in a constant state of chaos.

Medical doctors have described variations of migraine. Common migraine mimics classic migraine symptoms but without the early warning visual and sensory disturbances. "Migraine equivalents" exhibit the symptoms and patterns of migraine but lack the headaches. Commonly found in children, this latter variant often is mistaken for appendicitis because of its accompanying fever, nausea, vomiting, and abdominal pain. "Abdominal migraine" also lacks the headache component and includes vomiting, nausea, diarrhea, and abdominal pain. Extremely rare migraine forms include hemiplegic and ophthalmoplegic. In both instances headaches are moderate and symptoms of muscle weakness and paralysis occur on one side of the head and body. Ophthalmoplegic migraines characteristically manifest double vision, eye muscle weakness or paralysis resulting in a drooping eyelid.

# ANATOMY OF A MIGRAINE

My clinical experience in treating headache patients during the past ten years has revealed another major triggering factor of the migraine headache. This common denominator is dural torque. The excitement materialized when correlating migraine symptoms with the understanding of how the cranium, dural membranes, cerebrospinal fluid, blood flow, dental and pelvic complex interrelate and function.

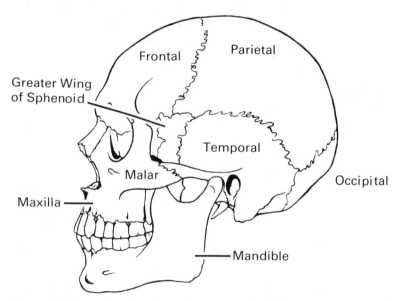

*Figure 5. The cranium is a dynamic structure that is in a constant state of micro-motion. This motion can occur because of the inherent flexibility of bone plus the presence of the expansion joints or sutures that lie between each bone. Architects design buildings, bridges, and roads with specific leeway for expansion, contraction and torsion. Nature, likewise provides for similar allowances in the flexibility of its hard and soft tissues and their interconnections.*

As previously described, the skull bones are inherently flexible. This flexibility comes from the fact that the cranial bones are saturated with blood and as stated in the textbook, *Gray's Anatomy,* bones derived from membrane (soft and flexible) will function like membrane throughout life. The bones that develop from membrane are those that make up the cranial vault (parietals, frontal, squama portion of the occipital and temporals, and greater wing of the sphenoid) (Fig. 5). Cranial bones are joined to one another by means of sutures. These sutures function like expansion joints. Architects and engineers design buildings, bridges, and roads with allowances for motion. For example, the Empire State and World Trade buildings in New York City each have a two foot sway, and bridges have a two inch leeway at either end to permit expansion, contraction and torquing. Why should the body, and more specifically, the architectural mastery of the cranium be any different?

To coordinate one side of the cranium to the other is the function of the dural membranes. These membranes are designed as vertical and horizontal tentpoles and have extensive attachments to the internal surfaces of the major cranial bones (Fig. 6). One source of head pain during a migraine attack comes from the internal pull of the dural attachment on the cranial sutural area. Another source of pain results from the engorged arteries and tension on the dural membranes themselves. All the membranes are themselves innervated and all twelve pairs of cranial nerves pass through at some point. The dural membranes also make up the extensive venous drainage system of the cranium. Of interest is the fact that the venous drainage out of the cranium occurs through foramina that are located in sutural areas between bones. The cranial bone motion surrounding the exiting vein serves as a pumping mechanism.

Eighty-five to 90 per cent of the venous (unoxygenated blood) drainage from the cranium occurs through the jugular vein. This vein exits by way of the jugular foramen which is located just anterior to the transverse process of the atlas (first cervical vertebra which joins with the base of the skull). Also exiting this jugular foramen are three major cranial nerves: glossopharyngeal (ninth), vagus (tenth), and accessory (eleventh).

*Figure 6. (See page 36.) The skull bones have reciprocal motion, i.e., when one side of the head is effected, the opposite side will automatically be involved. This action—reaction phenomenon occurs because of the extensive internal dural membrane attachments. These attachments are innervated by sensory nerves and in addition all the cranial nerves will pierce these membranes at some point. Distortions from whatever source will be transmitted throughout the dural membrane system. The appropriate sensory and motor portions of the brain will be activated to bring about the necessary structural and physiologic changes.*

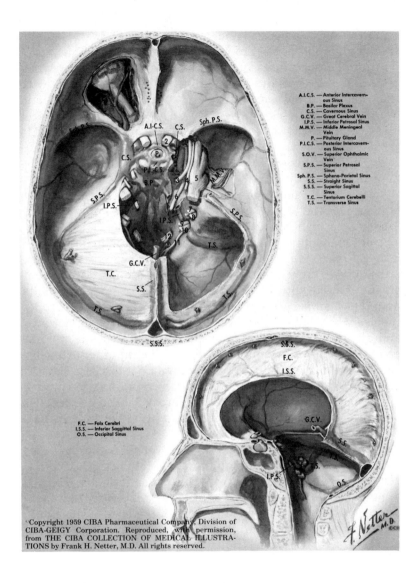

A.I.C.S. — Anterior Intercavernous Sinus
B.P. — Basilar Plexus
C.S. — Cavernous Sinus
G.C.V. — Great Cerebral Vein
I.P.S. — Inferior Petrosal Sinus
M.M.V. — Middle Meningeal Vein
P. — Pituitary Gland
P.I.C.S. — Posterior Intercavernous Sinus
S.O.V. — Superior Ophthalmic Vein
S.P.S. — Superior Petrosal Sinus
Sph. P.S. — Spheno-Parietal Sinus
S.S. — Straight Sinus
S.S.S. — Superior Sagittal Sinus
T.C. — Tentorium Cerebelli
T.S. — Transverse Sinus

F.C. — Falx Cerebri
I.S.S. — Inferior Saggittal Sinus
O.S. — Occipital Sinus

Copyright 1959 CIBA Pharmaceutical Company, Division of CIBA-GEIGY Corporation. Reproduced, with permission, from THE CIBA COLLECTION OF MEDICAL ILLUSTRATIONS by Frank H. Netter, M.D. All rights reserved.

*During a tension/or migraine headache, the muscles of the shoulders and back of the neck tighten up. The skull bones become pressed together in the sutural areas and create internal tensions within the dural membranes surrounding the brain. The dural tension created has the potential of causing far reaching neurological dysfunction. Any technique that will relieve muscle and dural tensions (manipulation, soft laser acupuncture, massage, rest, nutritional supplements, etc.) will effectively lessen the severity of the headache.*

The three cranial nerves exiting the jugular foramen have extensive innervations to many vital body areas. The glossopharyngeal nerve supplies taste and sensations to the posterior one-third of the tongue and throat. Neurological dysfunction of this nerve has the potential to cause loss of taste at the posterior one-third of the tongue, loss of the gag reflex, difficulty in swallowing, numbness to the throat, and increased salivation. The vagus nerve has extensive innervations with many important organs: larnyx (voice box), heart, lungs, stomach, liver, spleen, kidneys, pancreas, small intestine, and one half of the large intestine. Potential neurological problems include:

1. Difficulty in speaking
2. Difficulty in swallowing
3. Heart spasms
4. Heart arrhythmias (disturbed beating of the heart)
5. Stomach spasms
6. Paralysis of the soft palate
7. Spasms of the throat and chronic hoarseness
8. Intestinal problems
9. Breathing problems
10. Salivary disorders

Dysfunction of the eleventh cranial nerve involves the cervical musculature and is responsible for neck muscle spasms. These muscle spasms serve to perpetuate the problem since the structures leaving the jugular foramen are constantly being affected.

The dural tube consists of the cranial dural tentpoles (horizontal and vertical membranes), outer membranes that surround the brain, and membrane (dura) that surrounds the spinal cord along its entire length. After the dura exits the skull via the foramem magnum (opening at the base of the skull), it attaches tenaciously to the first three cervical vertebrae (atlas, axis, and C-3). Continuing down the spine, the dura terminates with its attachment to the sacrum (Fig. 1a and 1c). The sacrum is a wedge-shaped bone located between the two pelvic bones (ilia) and attached by means of strong ligaments.

The migraine sufferer is plagued by severe head pain and symptoms that affect half the body and may even switch sides during the course of an attack. The mystery of the migraine ceases once the concept of the dural tube torquing is understood (Fig. 7). As dental occlusion or structural misalignment of the pelvis, spinal vertebrae, or cranial bones occurs, a torquing pattern is set up in the system. Harry S.Truman aptly described the severity of a situation by stating that the buck stopped at the top! Similarly, the cranium is where the torque stops because it cannot go any further. Migraine sufferers have inherent structural weaknesses which predispose them to dural torquing. These predispositions can stem from distorted craniums, dental malocclusions, chronic muscle spasms (will cause distortions to the bony structures to which they are attached) spinal or pelvic anomalies. Every time a migraine episode occurs these victims experience the full-blown effects of structural imbalances.

The dominos begin to fall once the dural torquing commences. Tension builds within the cranial dural membranes placing pressure on those nerves within its path. As the torquing increases, the cranial bones are pulled in on one side more than the other. This distortion pattern becomes obvious in light of the fact that the cranial tentpoles provide a reciprocal tension membrane system. As one side tightens, the other side must reciprocate by relaxing. Cranial compensations accompanied by sutural jamming will invariably cause painful and tender areas to appear on the scalp.

As the structural distortions progress, the dural pressures will begin to retard the flow of cerebrospinal fluid (CSF) into the brain tissue. The beginning visual symptoms result from the visual centers of the brain being deprived of their normal quantities of blood and cerebrospinal fluid. As toxic metabolic wastes accumulate, neurological dysfunctions begin to abound. Increased cranial distortions will cause excess stimulation of the parasympathetic portion of the nervous system. Such stimulation has been documented to cause an increase in production of cerebrospinal fluid from the ventricles of the brain. The potential for an increased intracranial pressure now exists. Reduced blood outflow will also greatly contribute to the increased cranial pressure. The chain of events that set off the dural torquing will cause the atlas vertebra to distort.

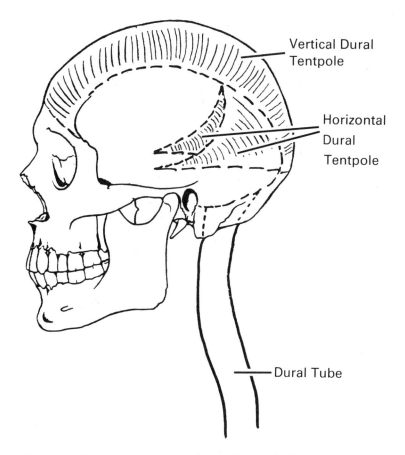

Vertical Dural Tentpole

Horizontal Dural Tentpole

Dural Tube

*Figure 7. Migraine headaches usually affect one-half of the victim's head. Since the dural tube is a reciprocating membrane, tension or torquing in the skull will cause one side to be in traction while the other side provides the slack. The nerves passing through the tensioned side will be responsible for the varied and extensive pains. The dural torquing can result from a single or various combinations of structural distortions such as the pelvis, spinal vertebrae, dental malocclusion or cranial bone restrictions. These structural problems can be triggered off by emotional, physical, nutritional or physiological stressors (e.g., organ dysfunction, under-active thyroid, muscle spasms or weakness, fixed and removable dental bridgework).*

This distortion occurs as a result of the firm dural attachment of the dural tube plus the fact that the atlas functions as a universal gear. In an attempt to reduce the tension on the cranial portion of the dural tube, the atlas will rotate out of position. Now the transverse process of the atlas unilaterally impinges on its anterior space. Occupying this anterior space and exiting the jugular foramen are the jugular vein, and ninth, tenth and eleventh cranial nerves. Tissue contracture and area swelling will cause a decreased blood flow out of the cranium further exacerbating the throbbing, pounding migraine headache. A true holistic approach will seek out major and compensatory structural imbalances and correct both. Upper cervical manipulation in conjunction with balancing total body mechanics will have the effect of releasing tensions, facilitating blood outflow and reducing nerve impingement.

Migraine symptoms relate primarily to structural, neurological, and physiological imbalances. When patients complain of facial pains involving half the face, invariably the pelvic complex is involved. Clinically, one ilium will be posteriorly rotated (associated with the functional short leg) while the other ilium will exhibit an anterior position (associated with the functional long leg). Because of the reciprocal dural tube interrelationships, the ilium and the temporal bones of the skull function in a synchronous arrangement. Other structures that follow this reciprocal relationship include the occiput and sacrum, sphenoid and coccyx, and the first three cervical and last three lumbar vertebrae respectively. These interrelationships follow Sir Isaac Newton's principle, "For every action there is an equal and opposite reaction." This reciprocal relationship holds true in approximately 90 per cent of the clinical cases involving subluxation or structural displacement patterns.

Of further interest is the fact that of twelve pairs of cranial nerves, nine pairs run in close proximity to the temporal bones. It is no wonder that structural distortion elicits such a wide spectrum of symptoms. The temporal bones are also of vital importance since they house the organs of balance. Dural torquing which distorts one temporal bone more than another has the potential to cause equilibrium problems and sensations of seasickness.

Symptom location provides an excellent indication of the source of imbalance. When patient complaints focus on midline head pains such as between the eyes or back midpoint of the head, vertebral distortions are usually the causative factor. Pains, paresthesias (abnormal sensations), pressures, and other symptoms that occupy one side of the cranium usually involve a pelvic distortion. Another rule of thumb regarding symptoms is that the farther away the symptom is from its source the greater the intensity of the symptom.

Weakness or paralysis of eye muscles usually involves the sphenoid bone and/or horizontal cranial tentpole (tentorium cerebelli). All but two of the muscles of the eye attach to the lesser wing of the sphenoid bone. Structural distortion of this bone will affect these muscles plus the horizontal membrane. Through this latter structure pass the four nerves (ophthalmic branch of the trigeminal [fifth cranial nerve], oculomotor [third cranial nerve] , trochlear [fourth cranial nerve], and abducens [sixth cranial nerve]) which innervate all the eye muscles.

Neurologically, the dura affects the central and automonic nervous systems. The latter system represents the involuntary portion of the nervous system and regulates our internal environment, such as the heartbeat, breathing, saliva flow, and digestion. This system also functions to provide for sudden alterations outside of the physiologic adaptive range. To accomplish this feat it operates in two parts: (1) the sympathetic portion, which supports the body when it is called into emergency action. It provides for increases in blood pressure, heart rate, breathing, slows digestion but increases blood sugar levels, and dilates the eye pupils causing sensitivity to light. (2) The parasympathetic system acts as a counterbalance to the sympathetic system and functions more to provide local changes. Parasympathetic dominance will cause such effects as an increase in stomach and intestinal secretions, contraction of the gallbladder, diarrhea, nausea, slowed heart rate and constriction of eye pupils with possible spasming of the muscles that control focus.

Structurally, the cranium and sacrum provide primarily parasympathetic stimulation while the thoracolumbar areas of the spine provide sympathetic nerve activity. The symptoms of migraine include blockage of nasal sinuses (histamine release), eye sensitivity to light (sympathetic dominance), nausea, vomiting, diarrhea and abdominal pains, all of which are related to overstimulation of the parasympathetic system. The resulting fever is due to the stored toxins which are normally released from the gallbladder into the intestinal track to be mixed and diluted with the passing food. Now, however, these toxins are dumped into an empty intestine and quickly absorbed into the bloodstream. The ensuing fever triggers mechanisms in the body to hasten its removal.

Continued parasympathetic activation will release several digestive enzymes (pepsin which digests protein and lipase which splits fats are the two most important) plus hydrochloric acid (HCL) within the stomach. The combination of pepsin and HCL functions as the "power" in breaking up protein. Overstimulation of the parasympathetic system will increase pepsin-HCL production. With little or no food in the stomach, this excess will cause nausea and irritation of the stomach lining resulting in abdominal pain and eventual ulceration. Vomiting is the quickest means by which the body's reflex mechanism can evacuate this irritant.

Pancreatic digestive enzymes plus bile from the gallbladder empty into the duodenum (first portion of the small intestine that connects to the stomach) to continue the digestive process. Parasympathetic stimulation from the cranium and/or sacrum also will release these enzymes. The combination of bile salts (which alone will cause diarrhea) plus all the liberated powerful digestive enzymes undiluted by food, presents the body with an extremely noxious and potentially dangerous situation. Because these substances are capable of digesting the small intestinal lining, the body reflexively evacuates these chemicals via the process of diarrhea.

## CRANIAL MIGRAINE

Sandra is a 43-year-old account executive who was referred by her psychologist for evaluation of post-whiplash symptoms. Prior to her motor vehicle accident, Sandra suffered from classic migraine headaches. In addition, she was sensitive to both alcohol and monosodium glutamate (MSG). Both substances would bring on violent headaches accompanied by nausea and vomiting. The physical trauma sustained in the automobile collision transformed the existing periodic headaches into a constant head pain, and in addition introduced the symptoms of frequent ringing noises in the left ear, dizziness, visual floaters, memory loss, and jaw clicking during chewing. Examination of the patient revealed extensive jamming of cranial sutures, restricted cranial bone ranges of motion, signs and symptoms of a weakened sacroiliac, and restricted cervical rotation and side bending movements. Palpation of her cranium revealed a disruption of both the primary and secondary cranial rhythms. There were also extensive spasms of the chewing muscles.

The patient was under the care of a chiropractor who had achieved a level of stability of the sacroiliac joint. My treatment consisted mainly of cranial manipulation to restore the cranial rhythms, release the sutural restrictions, and increase the ranges of motion. One week following the first cranial correction, the patient experienced tremendous relief. The headaches were completely gone, the ringing in the left ear was completely resolved, the dizziness was greatly reduced, her memory improved, and the visual eye floaters were also greatly diminished.

## PELVIC MIGRAINE

Edmond, a 35-year-old customer service representative came to my office in desperation. He admitted suicidal tendencies which stemmed from the severe headaches and body pain he had endured for the past 20 years.

In 1966 Edmond began experiencing headaches while in the armed services. These head pains appeared primarily on the left side of the head in the temporal bone area above the ear. In late 1969 he began experiencing severe cervical pain primarily on the right side. Between 1969 and 1974 the severity of the headaches increased along with upper cervical and lower back pains. By 1974 the intensity of the pains provoked thoughts of suicide. All diagnostic testing was negative. A neurosurgeon presented Edmond with the prognosis that future surgery would be necessary to correct the progressive paralysis. He was placed on the drug, Motrin, for the pain. A consulting orthopedic surgeon attributed the pains to cervical trauma and instituted cortisone injections into the symptomatic area of the cervical spine. Additional medical consultations elicited no further clues. The last consultation performed by a neurologist at the University of

Pennsylvania suggested that Edmond's problem was psychosomatic.

When Edmond presented himself for evaluation at my office, the entire left side of his body was affected with tingling and mild pain. He was experiencing severe deep pains in the upper right cervical area and entire left hemisphere of the skull. His neck and shoulders were always tight. Every morning he spent at least 15 minutes taking a hot shower to increase mobility of his neck and shoulders. He took ten milligrams of Valium daily prior to bedtime, Zantac, for occasional stomach pains, and 12 aspirins a day (which probably caused the stomach problem) for his headaches.

Clinically, the patient presented with a chronic sacroiliac weakness in which the left pelvic bone was posteriorly rotated causing a functional short leg. An interesting observation was that the patient always carried his wallet in his left pants pocket. The moderately thick billfold had the effect of further rotating the pelvis posteriorly greatly exacerbating the structural problem. Needless to say, he no longer carries his wallet in that pocket. Dentally, Edmond had a deep overbite and retruded lower jaw, both caused by the loss of several molar teeth. The cervical vertebrae exhibited restricted rotational and side-bending motions as compensations for both the dental malocclusion and sacroiliac weakness. Except for the torqued dural tube, the cranium presented only minor compensatory restrictions.

Exceptional results were achieved with the initial treatment. Utilizing the techniques discovered by Dr. DeJarnette, Edmond's pelvis was structurally corrected by padded wedges judiciously placed under each pelvic bone. This non-invasive, atraumatic approach permits the body's own weight to correct the distortion. The patient was instructed to place an ice bag over the sacroiliac area for 15 to 20 minutes every 5 hours for the next three days. This is designed to help reduce the inflammation in the joint area. During the following visit the patient informed me of tremendous reduction in both the cervical and the headache pain. He was able to reduce his aspirin intake from 12 to just two per day and the Valium was reduced by half to 5 mg. At the second visit, dental support was provided by bonding resins on the biting surfaces of the back teeth. This procedure was designed not only to reestablish a physiologic jaw posture but to stabilize the cervical vertebrae, dural tube, and sacroiliac joint.

As a patient, one must always be cognizant of the fact that when a structural problem exists no amount of drugs or surgical intervention will solve the problem. When a structural problem exists, correction can come only from manipulative techniques that focus on stabilizing the entire body.

## DENTAL MIGRAINE

Mary L. is a 38-year-old restaurant hostess who had suffered migraine headaches for the past twelve years. In 1980 the patient came to my office seeking help. Mary was at the end of her rope. She was addicted to Valium and pain killers. The drug effects were short-lived and she was getting desperate. She was also plagued with cervical and lower back pains which were getting progressively worse.

A severe dental malocclusion existed. Mary had lost a few molar and bicuspid teeth through the years. The remaining posterior teeth never fully erupted and she had a receded lower jaw. As a hostess she developed a few bad habits along the way. Mary would always cup the telephone between her shoulder and ear, and she invariably would bite on the end of her pen or pencil during her telephone conversations. Also, a poor diet which included numerous cups of coffee, donuts and other refined carbohydrates throughout the day raised havoc with her blood sugar level.

Treatment focused on reducing the quantity of caffeine, sugar, and other refined foods being consumed. The headaches, neck and lower back pains, diminished tremendously once dental support was provided by the fabrication of a lower partial denture. The appliance was physiologically designed to support the head and cervical vertebrae posture. Dental stability released the cranial and cervical torquing of the dural tube thus permitting the musculature to establish proper balance, and the cerebrospinal fluid to better circulate within the brain and restore neurological function.

# SCARRING, MUSCLE SPASMS, AND HEADACHES

In December 1985, Mary S. had surgery for the removal of a small tumor. The lump was located in a saliva gland just beneath her lower jawbone on the left side of her face. Prior to the operation, Mary had a few mild symptoms which included an occasional shooting pain up the left side of her face, which stopped over her left eye, mild pains on the back left side of her head and upper portion of the neck, mild left ear pains, and a moderate hearing loss of one year duration in the left ear that was discovered after a hearing test. Soon after the operation, all of Mary's symptoms worsened to the point that the pains became severe, constant, and unbearable.

Mary S. had been wearing full upper and lower dentures for the past 18 years. The lower denture fit poorly, irritated her lower gums and presented a major problem in chewing. In March of 1986, Mary had a consultation regarding the insertion of a lower dental implant which would stabilize the lower denture and improve chewing. The consulting crown and bridge specialist, Dr. Anthony Rinaldi, recognized that Mary's pain problem had some relationship to a structural imbalance of her jaw, neck and head. Dr. Rinaldi referred Mary for evaluation.

When Mary presented herself for examination at my office, she was experiencing severe pains in the left ear, left side of the jaw and face, and left side of the upper neck and base of the head. After examination, it was determined that Mary's problems stemmed from a distortion of her upper cervical vertebrae, muscle spasms, scar adhesions, and loss of a proper bite.

Because Mary S. lived out of state and travel time was extensive, treatment was started at the first visit. In order to resolve the muscle spasms and release the tissue tightness created by the four-inch scar, a nonsurgical soft laser beam was used on related acupuncture points, the actual scar, and the spastic muscles in the neck and facial areas. Within minutes after using the painless soft laser, the pains were completely erased, the muscle spasms began releasing, and Mary instantly regained her hearing in the left ear. The conductive hearing loss was due to a spastic muscle that controlled the opening of the left eustacian tube (tube that equalizes pressure between the middle ear and back of the throat) as well as of muscles that balance the tensions on the eardrum. In addition, gentle soft tissue release methods (myofascial techniques) were used to ease the neck tightness. These procedures were followed by gentle cranial manipulation to balance the cranial rhythm, release tensions in the cranial membranes, and free up the micro–motion between the cranial bones. To improve dental support and help maintain the structural balance that was achieved, the lower denture was built up with a soft lining material. Mary left the office completely out of pain and with her hearing restored.

Scars are one of the body's repair mechanisms for self healing. As the cut or torn tissues begin mending, the healing tissues knit a tight weave of fibers. The tightness of the scar has a local pulling effect on the muscles and also influences the entire elastic fibrous covering (fascia) that surrounds all body parts from head to toe. An example of fascial tension can be easily visualized by the motions of a nylon stocking in action on one's leg. The fine nylon filaments in a weave pattern provide flexibility to the stocking similar to the fascia of the body. If the stocking is pulled tightly at the top, an equal tension must occur somewhere else. The body's fascia acts no differently. In most people, the tensions are subtle and not sensed. However, if the scar is located over an organ, over a vital nerve area, or in individuals who have other structural imbalances, scars have the potential to worsen existing symptoms or cause new ones like headaches.

Dr. John E. Upledger, an internationally known researcher and lecturer in the field of cranial osteopathy, successfully treated a 36-year-old female patient who had suffered migraine headaches for 20 years. During the examination, Dr. Upledger discovered an abdominal restriction. Upon questioning, the patient gave a history of an appendectomy at age 12. Menstruation began at age 13; however, the headaches did not start until age 16. As with many patients, this woman visited many reputable clinics, exhausted most conventional therapeutic treatments, and was in the process of accepting her incapacitating migraines as the result of a deep-seated, psychoneurotic disorder. While examining the scar, it was discovered that placing deep, medial pressure on the scar produced the headache and deep lateral pressure brought headache relief.

The tensions within the scar tissue were released by treating with deep but gentle pressures. The patient remained headache-free during the 18 months following therapy and the publication of the report. In addition, following treatment of the scar, the woman experienced spontaneous relief of low back pain, menstrual disorders, and chronic and recurrent cervical problems.

At first glance, unconventional and unorthodox methods may seem bizarre and farfetched to the layperson and to many health professionals who have not opened their minds to such wisdom. On the other hand, the American public is unaware of the fact that only 10 to 20 per cent of all orthodox procedures currently used in medical practice have been shown to be effective by controlled experiment. This information appeared in an article entitled "Assessing the Efficacy and Safety of Medical Technologies" (Office of Technology Assessment, Publication #PB286-929, p.7, Sept. 1978). Skepticism on the part of highly trained physicians to accept that which is different stems from the present day medical model which is practically terrorized by so called analytical science. Doctors have become blind to elementary clinical observation which they label as subjective. One of America's great researchers on stress, the late Dr. Hans Selye, aptly described such judgmental insecurities when he stated, "If I throw a rock out of a window and it goes up instead of down, I don't need a double-blind study to prove that it's statistically significant."

# LASER THERAPY

For over fifteen years, actinotherapy, the therapeutic use of light, has been commonly used with great success in Europe. Because of its great therapeutic benefit, the nonsurgical helium--neon laser has been introduced into the United States. The ultra-low power (1 milliwatt) cold laser (also referred to as soft laser) is being used primarily for the reduction of acute and chronic pain, elimination of muscle spasms as well as enhancement of tissue healing.

The actual way in which laser light works has not yet been determined. One theory, however, explains the healing phenomenon in terms of a "biologic field." According to the Soviet scientist and originator of the theory, A.G. Gurvich, an energy field exists around all living cells, tissues and organs. The entire body as a whole influences the various organs of our body, which in turn influence the surrounding tissues. When an area is not functioning properly, the energy level is lower in that particular area. Directing the laser beam into acupuncture points as well as into the affected area will raise the energy level and help the body to resume normal function.

Presently, Germany, the Soviet Union, and the United States are engaged in clinical evaluation on laser safety. To date, all preliminary reports reveal that use of the ultra-low power laser has no harmful effects on living tissue when utilized properly. Testing indicates the intensity of these soft lasers to be equivalent to forty per cent of the intensity of a 100-watt light bulb, when the center of the bulb is held four inches from the skin. With virtually no heat output from the laser, living tissue will not become dehydrated or experience damage.

Because of the exceptional research and clinical successes in pain control by Joseph Kleinkort, a physical therapist in San Antonio, Texas, the United States military has adopted use of laser therapy. At present, lasers are in use at the Wilfordhall Air Force Base and the Walter Reed Army Medical Center in Washington, D.C. Through Mr. Kleinkort's lectures and workshops, many physicians and other healthcare practitioners are making laser therapy more accessible to the public.

Preliminary research findings show laser therapy to be beneficial in wound healing, migraine and vascular headaches, reduction of localized pain and inflammation of arthritis, shingles, muscle spasms, tendonitis, bursitis, postherpetic pain, and reduction in pain and swelling in patients suffering with rheumatoid arthritis.

The following case study was reported by Joseph Kleinkort, M.A., P.T. (4499 Medical Drive, Suite 380, San Antonio, TX.) and Russell A. Foley, B.S., P.T. in a published article, *Laser: A Preliminary Report on Its Use in Physical Therapy.* Clinical Management 2:32, 1983.

S.J., a 32-year-old white male, married, was in a state of good health until September 21, 1977. The patient was holding on to the boom of a heavy crane which came in contact with a high power line of approximately 220 volts of electricity. He was immediately rendered unconscious for approximately 90 minutes. The patient was hospitalized with electrical burns involving the chest and both upper arms. In addition, the patient presented with right upper arm paralysis. Numbness and impairment gradually resolved in three to four weeks.

The patient was initially seen on March 21, 1982 with complaints of severe headaches. The headaches occurred daily, were dull and steady in nature and increased in severity to a point that the patient became socially reclusive.

The patient described the headaches as burning in nature with a diffuse, throbbing and radiating pain from the neck region to the top of the head. The patient also complained of mild sensitivity to light, nausea, and vomiting. In response, the patient would retire to a quiet, dark room and pull the covers over his head.

All medical tests including CAT scans, myelograms, and neck and skull X-rays were normal. The patient was taking Clinoril and approximately four Empirin III and four Percodan tablets per day, which provided only minor relief. In addition, Fiorinal, Valium, Motrin, Indocine and Parafon Forte had been ineffective in bringing any relief of the symptoms.

The patient was started on a series of laser treatments to the neck and various other acupuncture points. A TENS (transcutaneous electrical nerve) unit was used for pain control. A detoxification program was used to clear out the medications from the body. Various physical therapy techniques were initiated to correct muscular restrictions in the neck, chest and upper arms.

Following a series of ten visits, the patient was totally free of all symptoms. The patient experienced no further headaches and required no medications. Significant improvement was noted in the patient's social life, to a point where he enjoyed an overall increased quality of life.

## Case Study

Gloria is a 49-year-old female who had been suffering upper left neck and shoulder aches and pains for over a year and a half. The injuries occurred while on duty as an undercover policewoman at a local hotel. While walking down a flight of padded stairs, Gloria reached for the railing for support. The railing, unfortunately, was not secured and pulled away from the wall causing Gloria to tumble down fourteen steps.

The orthopedic examination and x-rays revealed no broken bones and all other diagnostic tests were negative. Gloria followed through with the initial drug therapy of muscle relaxers and pain killers; however she could not function because of the drowsiness caused by the medication. The next step involved physical therapy in the form of heat packs, ultrasound, transcutaneous electrical nerve stimulation (TENS), muscle massage and joint mobilization techniques. Although some temporary relief occurred, Gloria still experienced pains and stiffness, especially when there was a change in the weather.

Gloria discontinued conventional treatment after six months because no lasting relief was achievable. At this point, Gloria gave up hope, resigned herself to the fact that she would have to live with the pain and was skeptical that she was ever going to recover from the injury. Approximately nine months elapsed when Gloria's sister-in-law told her about the benefits she had received from soft laser therapy. Although somewhat skeptical of obtaining any major cure, Gloria set up an appointment.

At her first appointment, Gloria made it clear that she came more out of curiosity about what her sister-in-law had told her than from the belief that she was really going to be helped. Because of the chronic muscle tightness, I employed osteopathic myofascial release techniques in conjunction with the soft laser. The first visit lasted about one hour, and Gloria left with minimal discomfort and a definite increase in neck mobility. Because the relief lasted longer than previous treatments, Gloria followed up with two additional one hour sessions approximately one month apart. At the end of that three-month period, all her symptoms had resolved, including the flare-ups that occurred with weather changes. Needless to say, Gloria's skepticism vanished quickly.

---

Dear Dr. Smith:

Thirteen months ago I was rear-ended while stopped at a traffic light. At first the impact seemed to be only a passing shock but then I felt a severe burning sensation shooting up by head and down my back.

During the eleven months following my accident I was treated by 13 different doctors and spent 9 days in the hospital in traction. All the medical tests kept coming up negative, but I still was in a lot of pain.

My life turned into a real nightmare. I couldn't even find a comfortable position let alone stay awake from the prescribed muscle relaxers.

In despiration, I began praying for someone to help me. My chiropractor, Dr. Cobb, took five of his patients, including myself, to have soft laser treatments by you.

Since those treatments, my headaches have disappeared and my body pains have been reduced tremendously. Now that I am getting better I feel I will again be able to live a more normal life. Thanks go first to God for giving me the strength to come through all the pain and suffering and second for giving you the knowledge to uncover this medical maze.

A grateful patient,

*Barbara S.*

Barbara S.

---

# AURICULOTHERAPY

This form of therapy was discovered back in the early 1950s by a French physician, Paul Nogier. Dr. Nogier's research uncovered the astonishing correlation of the structure of the ear to that of the rest of the human body. When visualized, the fetus' body can be projected onto the auricle (Figure 8). The head is situated at the bottom of the ear while the hands and feet can be found at the top of the auricle. Not only is the shape similar but every point of the body has a corresponding ear point. These corresponding points are noticeable only when palpated and the individual is not healthy. During the initial stages of dysfunction, localized sore spots will be present on the ear. As the body becomes more chronically ill, specific projections will appear and become painful.

Looking at the ear closely, one sees that it is shaped exactly like a human embryo and in essence represents a microcosm of the whole body. Acupuncturists consider the ear one of the most important parts of the human body. As noted in the third diagram, the ear contains tiny acupuncture points which correspond to every part and organ in the body.

The connection between the ear and the various body parts is explained by the extensive innervation of the ear and the multiple connections with the central nervous system. This interrelationship provides the basis for auriculotherapy. As stated by Dr. Nogier, "The ear is both a dashboard and a control center by means of which the illness can be treated."

Therapy is applied by means of physical agents, e.g., massage, acupuncture, electrical stimulation, and cauterization. This author has expanded on Dr. Nogier's original work by utilizing soft laser in combination with galvanic stimulation (therapeutic use of direct current). The results have been tremendous.

Use of soft laser on the auricular points has been very effective especially in treating patients with acute and chronic muscle spasm pain. The post-trauma patient is frequently

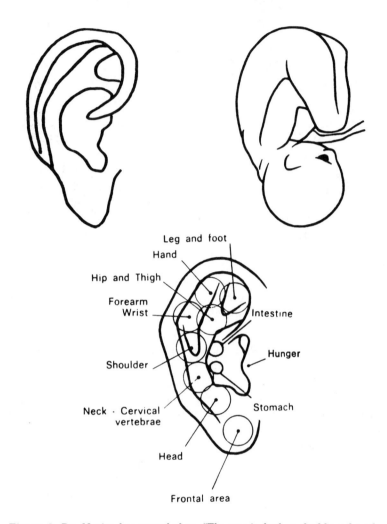

*Figure 8. Dr. Nogier has stated that, "The ear is both a dashboard and a control center by means of which the illness can be treated." Every major body area, including the brain and organs, has an acupuncture ear point.*

plagued by such suffering. Victims of whiplash injuries, falls, sprains and strains, and TMJ related muscle pain respond well to auriculotherapy. Laser treatment is remarkable in that the acute pains are often alleviated almost immediately. In those cases in which the pain pattern was not completely resolved, the severity of the pain was lessened to a great degree.

## Case Study 1

Anna, a 66-year-old practical nurse, was involved in a motor vehicle accident. The car in which she was a passenger was struck from the rear. As a result of the impact, Ann's head hit the inside roof of the car. Immediately following the injury, Anna began suffering with frontal headaches, bilateral neck pains, right shoulder pain, shooting pains across and down her lower back and along her right leg. In addition, she experienced symptoms of "jawlash" which included painful jaws and bilateral pains in the temporal areas.

Treatment focused on a combination of galvanic stimulation in conjunction with soft laser acupuncture. Specific points on Anna's ear, upper neck, hand, TMJ, and painful muscle trigger points were stimulated. The patient experienced immediate relief of pain and increased mobility of her neck. When Anna returned two weeks later for follow-up therapy, she stated that her headaches were completely gone, the shooting pains across and down her back and right leg were gone and that she never felt better.

## Case Study 2

Esther came to my office seeking relief from upper back pains which resulted from a fall. While shopping in a local supermarket, Esther reached for a product on an upper shelf. There was a puddle of water in the immediate area and before she realized it her feet went out from under her. On the way down, she apparently struck two shelves causing trauma to her back about the level of the upper portion of the shoulder blades. In addition, the left leg and knee were injured. As a result of her inability to function without pain, Esther could no longer perform her duties as a dance instructor.

Conventional drug therapy and physical therapy were used by previous doctors, but to no avail. Esther was also tired of taking the pain killers and muscle relaxers. The medication not only failed to relieve the pain but made her too drowsy to function. Even though her problem was chronic and lasted over a year, immediate relief resulted from the first soft laser treatment. As with previous pain patients, all the associated acupuncture points were treated. By the third treatment session, the patient's pain pattern had been reduced enough for her to begin slowly working out to get back in shape so that she could resume teaching dance.

It is this author's opinion that traditional medicine has reached its peak of sophistication. The advances in chemotherapy, exotic surgery, and new generation computer assisted tomography (CAT) scans have brought tremendous changes to the healing arts. The next phase within the healing professions will witness utilization of laser acupuncture therapy, cranial and structural manipulation, electromedicine, nutritional support, and a return to more natural eating habits as the principal means of restoring and maintaining health.

# Part III

# A New Specialty Is Born

# PHYSIOLOGIC DENTISTRY

A grassroots movement has been developing within the ranks of the dental profession within the past thirty years. These professionals represent the pioneers in a field that has gone beyond the parameters of drilling and filling teeth, treating gum disease, extracting teeth, fabricating mechanical replacements for missing teeth, and teaching plaque control. As creative thinkers, these men have painstakingly linked various medical problems to a common dental origin–malocclusion. Researchers like Drs. Nathan Shore, Willie May, Harold Gelb, Alred Fonder, Harold Ravins, Stephen Smith, Carl Mestman, Justine Jones and many others have discovered the significance of the patient's bite and its relationship to the rest of the body. Proper tooth alignment and bite helps establish:

1. a psysiologic muscle length for the chewing muscles as well as those of the throat, neck, and shoulder.

2. a self-correcting mechanism for balancing cranial bones.

3. sufficient vertical forces into the cranium which aid the pumping mechanism in distributing cerebrospinal fluid around and into the entire brain.

4. proper head, neck, shoulder, spinal and pelvic posture.

5. stability of the sacroiliac joint and pelvic complex.

6. normal blood and lymphatic flow in the head and neck.

7. adequate blood and oxygen supply to the brain.

8. neurologic balance of the sympathetic and parasympathetic nervous systems.

9. structural equilibrium of the organs of balance.

10. a patent airway within the eustachian tube (connects the middle ear and throat).


## STRESS AND DISTRESS


A malocclusion presents the body with a constant structural imbalance which translates into a state of distress. As defined by Dr. Hans Selye, distress always refers to an activity that is damaging. In 1936 Dr. Selye discovered the general adaptation syndrome in which all stressors such as physical, chemical, or psychological damaging agents will provoke a reproducible nonspecific body response. Although his original experiments were conducted on laboratory animals, the exact results have since been verified in humans. The body's defense system provides a three-tier reaction :

1. **Alarm stage:** The body exhibits characteristic changes resulting from exposure to the stressor. The body's nonspecific reactions involve a three phase response. First, the adrenal cortex (outer layer that produces hormones such as cortisone) becomes hyperactive and enlarges. Second, the thymus gland and lymphatic tissue shrink (these tissues relate to the body's immune system). Last, gastrointestinal ulcers appear.

2. **Resistance stage:** Body resistance will follow if continued exposure to the stressor (malocclusion for example) results in adaptation. The signs of the alarm stage will disappear and resistance will be maintained.

3. **Exhaustion stage:** Long-term exposure to the same stressor, to which the body had previously adapted, will deplete the stores of adaptation energy. The signs of the alarm stage will reappear, may become irreversible, and if the individual or body fails to eliminate the causative factors, death usually results.

Selye defined stress as a state within the body which produces observable symptoms, not just vague or general nervous tension. It was Selye's contention that each of us tends to respond to stress with a particular set of signs. He believed that when these signs appear it is nature's way of telling us to change our activity and find diversion. The following is a list of self-observable signs of stress:

1. General irritability, hyperexcitation or depression
2. Pounding of the heart
3. Dryness of the throat and mouth
4. Impulsive behavior; emotional instability
5. The overpowering urge to cry or run and hide
6. Inability to concentrate
7. Feelings of unreality, weakness, or dizziness
8. Predilection to become fatigued
9. "Floating anxiety" (being afraid but not knowing exactly of what)
10. Emotional tension and alertness; feeling of being keyed up
11. Trembling; nervous tics
12. Tendency to be easily startled by small noises
13. High-pitched nervous laughter
14. Stuttering and other speech difficulties which are stress induced
15. Bruxism, clenching or grinding of the teeth
16. Insomnia
17. Hyperkinesia (increased tendency to move about without any reason)
18. Sweating
19. Frequent need to urinate
20. Diarrhea, indigestion, queasiness in the stomach, and sometimes even vomiting
21. Migraine headaches
22. Premenstrual tension or irregular menstrual cycles
23. Pain in the neck or lower back due to muscle tension
24. Loss of or excessive appetite
25. Increased smoking
26. Increased use of legally prescribed drugs
27. Alcohol or drug addiction
28. Nightmares
29. Neurotic behavior
30. Psychoses
31. Accident proneness

The body reacts to any and all types of influences by entering a state of stress. Whether distortions of the cranial, dental or pelvic complex, physiologic or psychologic dysfunctions exist, the three stages of symptoms are specific as mentioned previously. As these stress-related responses go beyond the physiologic adaptive range of the body's ability to cope, a transition into distress occurs with clinical manifestations.

## DENTAL DISTRESS SYNDROME (DDS)

Patients who have been labeled as hypochondriacs often suffer from the *dental distress syndrome.* Dr. Fonder has stated that "DDS is produced by maloccluded teeth (Figs. 9a and 9b) and the resultant spasms and malfunctioning of the musculature of the jaws, head, neck, and shoulders routinely cause pathological alterations throughout all systems of the body and mind." Many of these patients complain of chronic

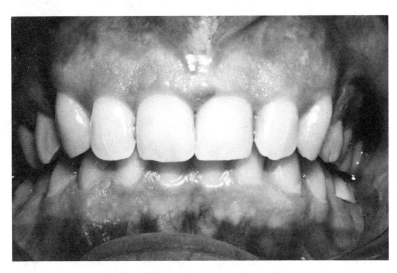

*Figure 9a. The deep overbite (loss of vertical posterior tooth support) represents one of the most common improper bites that cause the dental distress syndrome. Loss of support from back teeth can have a genetic factor or may come from premature loss of teeth, lack of adequate eruption, normal wearing down of the chewing surfaces of either dentures or natural teeth, clenching and grinding one's teeth (bruxism), dental equilibration (grinding of the chewing surfaces by a dentist to correct an improper meshing of teeth), extraction of bicuspid teeth for orthodontic treatment, and intrusion of teeth due to prolonged use of a TMJ orthopedic appliance.*

headaches (including migraine), dizziness, hearing loss, depression, eye pains, facial pains, anxiety, nervousness, forgetfulness, chronic fatigue, insomnia, sinusitis, indigestion, frequent urination, stomach ulcers, dermatitis, allergies, kidney and bladder complications, cold hands and feet, vague and distinct body pains and numbness, suicidal tendencies, sexual failures, and gynecological problems.

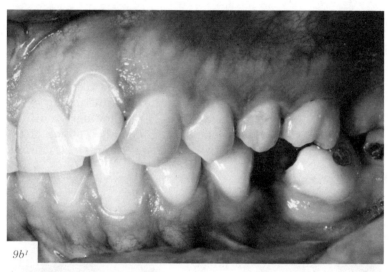

9b¹

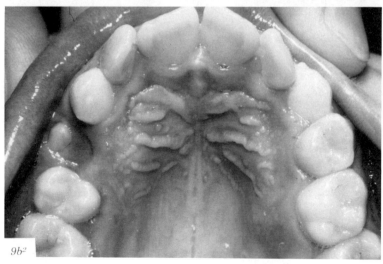

9b²

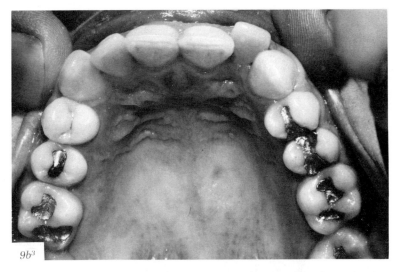

9b³

*Figure 9b. The retruded lower jaw represents another malocclusion that has the potential to distort body posture.( 9b¹ ) Dental structural distortions of this form are usually caused by either a narrow upper jaw ( 9b² ) or backward tilting of the upper front teeth.( 9b³ )*

*All dental malocclusions have the potential, to varying degrees, to alter total body functioning. Some areas directly affected include the cranium, chewing muscles, neck vertebrae, spine, pelvis, nervous system, immune system, digestive system and psychological performance of the individual.*

Dr. Al Fonder clinically observed and documented a host of structural body distortions routinely associated with an improper bite:

1. Lateral spinal curvature (scoliosis)
2. Forward spinal curvature (lordosis)
3. Humpback or backward spinal curvature (kyphosis)
4. Pelvic rotation
5. Uneven shoulder height
6. Side head tilt and forward head posture
7. Displaced organ position due to skeletal structural distortions
8. Reduction of blood, oxygen, and lymphatic flow in the head and neck

Dr. Fonder also observed clinically that removal of the dental distress allowed the body, in many cases, to self-correct–structurally, chemically, and psychologically (Figs. 10a, 10b, and 10c).

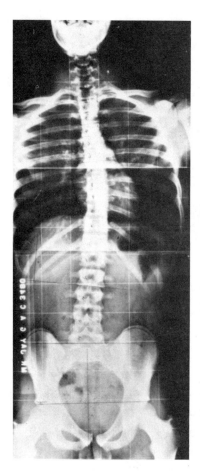

*Anteroposterior view before treatment.*

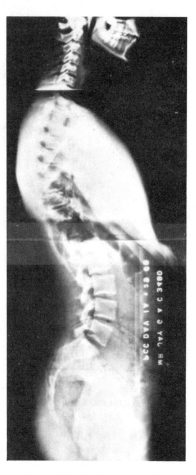

*Lateral view before treatment.*

**Figure 10a.** *The before and after radiographs represent those of a 16-year-old boy who had a malocclusion. Dr. Fonder restored the boy's bite by adding 1/2 mm additional height by means of an amalgam filling material on the lower second molar teeth. The after treatment x-rays reveal a definite decrease in the lateral spine (scoliosis) and backward bend spinal curvature distortions.*

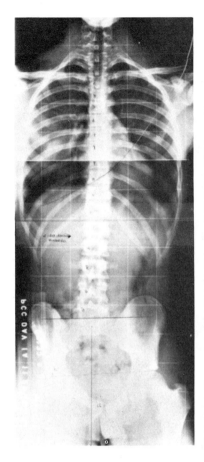

*Anteroposterior view after treatment.*

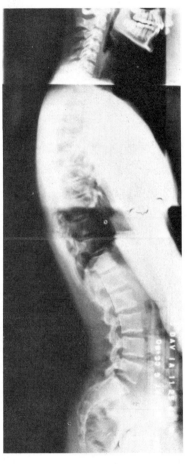

*Lateral view after treatment.*

65

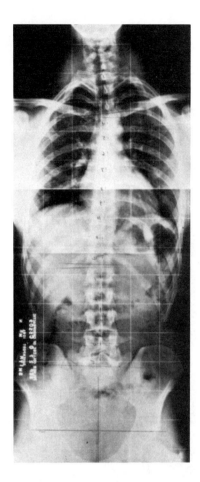

*Anteroposterior view before treatment.*

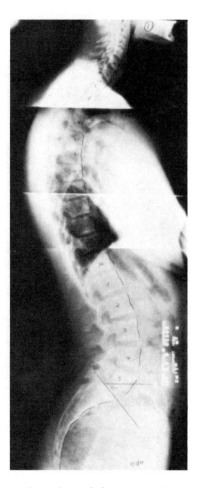

*Lateral view before treatment.*

***Figure 10b.*** *A 21-year-old student presented with a deep overbite malocclusion accompanied by an inward tilting of the upper and lower back molar and bicuspid teeth. Also present was a structural spinal misalignment in the form of a scoliosis and kyphosis (humpback). Treatment utilized upper and lower dental orthopedic expansion appliances which uprighted the back teeth and raised the jaw height. The before and after x-rays reveal the changes that took place.*

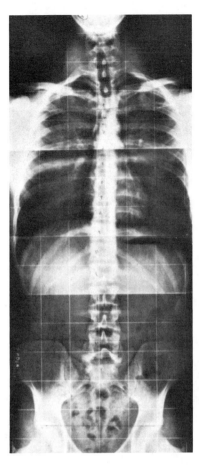

*Anteroposterior view after treatment.*

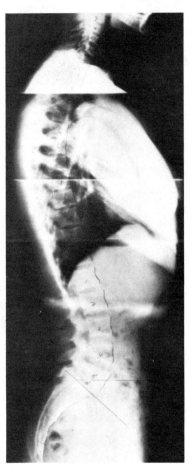

*Lateral view after treatment.*

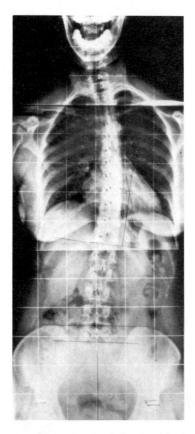

*Anteroposterior view before treatment.*

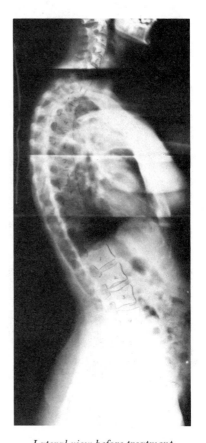

*Lateral view before treatment.*

*Figure 10c. This chronically ill and despondent homemaker presented the following chief complaints: severe headaches, intense backaches, difficulty in negotiating stairs, balance problems, blurred vision, hearing loss, gastrointestinal problems, gynecological disturbances accompanied by severe premenstrual cramps. The headaches caused her to spend many days in bed. The backaches prevented her from raising her arms above the shoulders. Because conventional therapy was unable to alter her symptoms, she was advised to seek psychiatric help. At one point, the woman contemplated suicide.*

*The patient's bite was "collapsed" as a result of several missing molar teeth. Treatment provided temporary fixed bridgework to replace the missing*

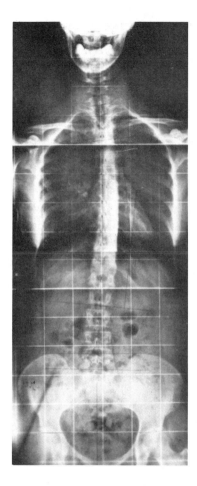

*Anteroposterior view after treatment.*

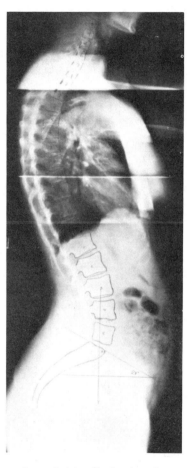

*Lateral view after treatment.*

posterior teeth. *The patient experienced immediate relief from the previous, constant neck tension. The day after treatment the woman was able to raise both arms above the shoulders, had no more balance problems, and was free of headaches and backaches. One week following treatment she was able to run up and down the stairs with no difficulty. The woman became so energetic that she took a job as a bridal consultant and was on her feet all day long for six days a week. The patient remained symptom-free because the structural imbalances had been corrected.*

**69**

Physiologic dentistry grew out of thousands of clinical observations like those made by Dr. Fonder. The honors must go to the small percentage of inquisitive and persistent dentists who had the courage to pursue their investigations. These pioneers noticed the disappearance of many medical problems once their patients' malocclusions were corrected.

## DENTAL "HATBAND" HEADACHE

One of the most frequent violations of the cranium occurs when conventional dental techniques restrict cranial bone motion by crossing the maxillary midline with fixed bridgework. Because each maxilla is connected to nine other cranial bones (malar, frontal, ethmoid, vomer, palatine, lacrimal, sphenoid, inferior nasal concha, and the other maxilla) it represents direct contact with 45 per cent of the cranium. In essence, locking the maxillae will restrict, to varying degrees, the entire craniosacral mechanism. Since each patient's physiologic adaptive range varies, the clinical extent of the symptoms will ultimately depend on the levels of distress. Patient complaints of severe headaches, facial pain, chronic fatigue, mental confusion, eye pains, irritability, disequilibrium and many more seemingly unrelated symptoms have been resolved once the midline restriction was removed and normal cranial rhythm reestablished.

## CASE STUDY

A 42-year-old female was referred to me for evaluation of numerous chronic symptoms. The dental history revealed extensive fixed upper bridgework fabricated by a board–certified prosthodontist. The patient's symptoms began after cementation of fourteen units of fixed upper bridgework and included a high fever for several days afterward. Some symptoms appeared immediately upon bridge placement while others were progressive. The permanent bridgework was completed fourteen months prior to my evaluation. The following chief complaints were presented by the patient:

1. Constant "hatband" headache–immediate
2. Facial and skull tightness–immediate
3. Generalized feeling of stress and irritability–immediate
4. Upper cervical neck pains–immediate
5. Limited right and left rotation of the head–immediate
6. Disequilibrium–progressive
7. Generalized chronic fatique–progressive
8. Generalized muscle weakness–progressive
9. Paresthesia (abnormal sensations) in the arms and legs–progressive

The patient's medical history at the time of examination was unremarkable. Her past medical history revealed only some minor surgery. The medical report revealed all of her systems to be essentially normal. A blood work-up showed all values to be within normal limits. Clinical examination revealed numerous tender sutural areas on the cranium, 45-degree rotational restriction of the head to the right and left, and a 20 per cent hearing loss in the low frequency range (125 and 250). Videofluoroscopic motion studies revealed a definite restriction of movement of the first two cervical vertebrae, primarily in flexion–extension positions.

The diagnosis made was dural torque. The cause was cranial restrictions stemming from the fixed bridgework. Emergency treatment was rendered by cutting the maxillary midline connection between the central incisor crowns (two front teeth). Immediate relief was felt as soon as the cast connection was separated. The "hatband" headache, facial and cranial tightness, head rotation restriction, upper cervical pain, cranial stress disappeared immediately. Within ten days the paresthesia in the arms and legs diminished such that only a slight residual effect remained in the right arm. In approximately two weeks, the remaining symptoms of disequilibrium, chronic fatigue, and muscle weakness resolved.

The hearing test conducted after the bridgework was cut revealed an increase of 20 decibels in the low frequency range (125 and 250). Since hearing was immediately restored to normal upon releasing the cranium via cutting the bridgework, it is apparent that the middle ear bone restriction was due to the restriction of the cranial bones. Post-treatment videofluoroscopic radiography revealed even more interesting results with an increase in flexion– extension movements of the head.

The question of whether cranial bone motion exists is no longer an issue. The issue now is how not to violate this physiologic motion when restoring the teeth. Cranial restrictions have far reaching effects on potentially the entire physiology of the body including cranial rhythm, flow of cerebrospinal fluid, blood flow, dural membrane torque, and pressure on cranial nerves, cervical vertebrae, and sacrum.

Similarly, patients who have partial upper dentures and are unable to tolerate the appliance for any length of time are victims of cranial bone restriction. The partial upper denture, especially if fabricated of a cast metal, is rigid and will restrict normal physiologic cranial motion.

**Case Study**

In 1980, Mike underwent full mouth dental reconstruction for the second time. Fifteen years previously, all his teeth had been capped. Wear and tear plus the loss of a few teeth due to gum disease necessitated redoing the existing bridgework. Because of missing upper posterior teeth bilaterally, a removable partial denture was constructed. The partial upper denture was retained by means of precision attachments which connected it to the remaining bridgework. The fit was like that of a surgical glove. Because of the rigid cast bar that spanned the roof of his mouth, the cranium was locked in position. Mike was unable to tolerate the appliance in his mouth for even a short time. The restriction of normal cranial motion created such an excess of neurological stress within his head that his body could not cope with the overload. The solution at the time was to discontinue wearing the appliance.

Today Mike's problem would be resolved easily through the use of a flexible resin material called Resiflex. This material is bonded along the midline of the partial upper denture to permit normal physiologic cranial motion. Individuals who have run into this problem can have their dentists purchase the material from ICNR, INC. (P.O. Box 55, Newtown, Pa. 18940).

# DENTAL MALOCCLUSIONS

Dental malocclusions present as either skeletal or dental problems. Skeletal problems develop from genetic factors. These are usually observed as discrepancies in jaw size. Problems of this nature must be dealt with through the use of dental orthopedics, surgery, or a combination of both. On the other hand, malocclusions of dental origin can be treated orthodontically by straightening the teeth or by the use of either removable appliances, such as partial dentures, or fixed crowns or bridgework.

Malocclusions are viewed as discrepancies in any one or any combination of three planes: vertical, horizontal or front to back. The majority of these problems stem from the "western civilized diet" consisting primarily of refined and processed foods. Drs. Price and Pottinger have documented these changes in recent generations of primitive people and have shown that in the span of just one generation the first offspring developed malocclusions when their parents were placed on a refined food diet. The lack of adequate minerals such as calcium, magnesium, zinc, manganese, etc., and the lack of unaltered protein, various vitamins, and dietary fiber prevents the dental arches from fully developing.

It has been my clinical experience that the greatest discrepancy exists in the vertical plane (deep overbite) and narrow width of the upper jaw (maxillae). Loss of jaw height is commonly described by the layperson as a deep overbite. Viewed dentally, the upper teeth overlap the lower teeth by three millimeters or more (Fig. 9a). The discrepancy may not seem like a major structural problem until one visualizes the entire structural interplay. A lack of vertical support will cause the jaw joint (temporomandibular joint) to move upward. As a result of this overclosure, the disc that normally sits on top of the jaw joint lacks sufficient space, becomes compressed, and eventually is displaced. Constant pressure generated over a period of time will cause wear and tear on the head of the joint, resulting in what is commonly referred to in medical jargon as osteoarthritis. Joint compression affects the nerves, blood supply, and lymphatics and causes micro-trauma to the joint tissues. As the upper and lower jaws come closer together, so do the muscles that are attached to the jaws.

Davis's Law now comes into play: "The shorter the length of the muscle, the stronger it becomes." As these muscles tighten up and become spastic, they pull harder on the bony structures to which they are attached. Those chewing muscles that are anchored on the cranium will greatly influence cranial motion, cranial sutures and dural membranes. Dr. DeJarnette has always taught, "Muscles affect bone, bone affects sutures, the sutures affect the dura and the dura influences the function of the brain." The chewing muscles that extend below the jaw will affect the shoulder girdle to which they are attached. Other muscles that attach from the shoulder girdle extend to the upper cervical vertebrae. Cervical distortions result in head postural problems, distortions of the lower lumbar vertebrae, changes within the spine and changes in the pelvic complex, which also reciprocates with the shoulder girdle. The nerves of the chest portion of the spine supply all the major organs of the body. Because of jaw misalignment, the receptors of the TM joint become activated along with all the other joint receptors of the body. They become functional to insure total structural balance. The seemingly insignificant loss of a few millimeters of jaw height sets off a domino effect that ultimately has the potential to involve the entire structural, neurological and physiological aspects of the body.

## DENTAL EAR CONNECTION

Over thiry years ago Dr. Fonder conducted a study which demonstrated that hearing loss and ear problems were related to malocclusion of the teeth. His initial pilot study demonstrated a definite hearing loss pattern in every malocclusion patient tested. A follow-up study involving 1500 children (3,000 consecutive ears tested) with dental malocclusions demonstrated a loss in hearing acuity in every individual tested.

Many anatomic relationships connect the functioning of the ear and the dental complex. The first involves a small ligament (Pinto's ligament) that extends from the medial pole of the jaw joint to the neck of one of the middle ear bones. The middle ear bones, or ossicles, transmit sound vibrations from the eardrum to the internal ear. Distortion of the jaw position has the potential to affect the transmission of vibrations over the ossicles and reduce hearing in the lower frequency range (Fig. 11). Hearing loss is not always apparent until after dental corrections re-establish jaw posture. Patients often remark that they are able to hear sounds not previously perceived.

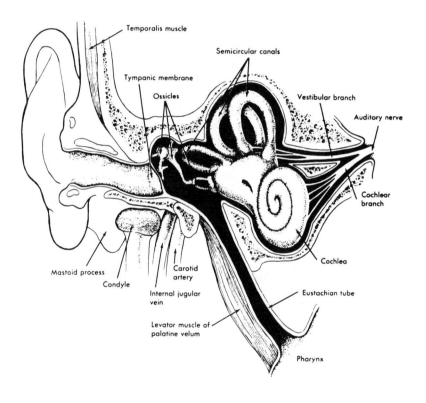

*Figure 11. The jaw joint lies in close proximity to the middle ear. Distortions of jaw position due to an improper bite, muscle spasms, or a retrusion of the jaw resulting from a whiplash injury has the potential to cause ear problems (ear noises—ringing, hissing, buzzing, conductive hearing loss, increased pressure, and pain).*

## Case Study 1

Eleanor is a 45-year-old nurse who noticed a progressive conductive hearing loss over the past several years. Initially Eleanor sought dental services to restore missing back teeth, as well as defective capping and decayed teeth. As posterior teeth were lost because of extensive caries, the bite began collapsing. One sequela of lost vertical jaw position involves the dysfunction of the oral musculature. Often affected is the tensor veli palatini muscle which governs the opening of the eustacian tube. The middle ear pressure is equalized during swallowing by the passage of air via the eustacian tube, from the throat to the middle ear. A spastic tensor veli palatini muscle or distorted temporal bone has the potential to restrict the opening of the eustacian tube thus preventing equal atmospheric pressure on both sides of the eardrum. Under such conditions, the inability of the ossicular chain and eardrum to vibrate effectively causes a conductive hearing loss.

Eleanor underwent extensive restorative dentistry which involved capping all her remaining upper teeth and constructing a partial lower denture. Upon completion of treatment, the patient had returned for a postoperative adjustment. During that visit Eleanor remarked that her hearing was better since her bite was restored with the fixed and removable partial lower appliance.

Another interesting anatomic relationship involves one of two muscles of the middle ear. The tensor tympani muscle originates from the sphenoid bone and extends to the malleus bone which attaches to the eardrum. The function of the two muscles is to prevent the middle ear bones from transmitting excessive noise. The lower jaw interrelates with the sphenoid bone via the external pterygoid muscle. It is this muscle that most often goes into spasm when there is a loss of jaw height. Spasm of this muscle will refer pain into the ear, mimicking an earache, and may cause many unsuspecting physicians to treat the patient's complaint with antibiotics and pain killers as if a middle ear infection existed. Spasm of this muscle will also distort the sphenoid bone, and in turn the tensor tympani will spasm, affecting the ossicular chain, reducing hearing, and possibly causing ear noises.

## Case Study 2

Muriel is a 34-year-old housewife who had been suffering severe left ear pain in addition to pain in her upper and lower left molar teeth. Visits to the family physician and to an ear, nose and throat (ENT) specialist ruled out the possibility of any infection or pathology. In desperation, Muriel presented herself to me for a dental evaluation to seek a possible cause for the pain. Radiographs of the teeth revealed no decay, and no broken fillings or abscesses. However, examination of the chewing muscles uncovered the presence of a severely painful upper left external pterygoid muscle. This muscle, which governs mouth opening and attaches from the head of the jaw joint (located in front of the ear) to the lateral pterygoid plate of the sphenoid bone, was in spasm. Spastic muscles always have trigger points ( small nodular extremely painful areas within the muscle) which refer pain to other areas. The referral pain pattern of this muscle includes the ear, and upper and lower molar teeth.

Resolution of Muriel's problem was relatively simple once the proper diagnosis was made. Treatment consisted of a technique called "strain, counter-strain." Finger pressure is applied to the painful trigger point while gently thrusting the head forward. This particular procedure is painful, but the relief is dramatic and immediate. Muriel left the office pain-free and very grateful.

## Case Study 3

At age 51, Louise suddenly became plagued by constant tinnitus. The constant ringing in her ears made it difficult for her to function. She was first treated by her family physician with antibiotics for a suspected middle ear infection. When the tinnitus did not clear up, Louise was referred to an ENT specialist who proceeded to drain fluid from her middle ear. The problem still persisted after all conventional methods of treatment failed.

When Louise presented herself for evaluation, her chief complaints were general fatigue, ear stuffiness, post-occipital headaches, sinus congestion, neck stiffness, and popping and clicking of the jaw joints. Dental evaluation revealed many missing posterior molar and bicuspid teeth. When consulted, her family dentist stated that the patient had been uncooperative in that she had never followed through with her proposed dental treatment. The patient expressed her reluctance to submit to any form of dental treatment that did not address itself to solving her problems. When presented with an approach to resolve her complaints, there was no hesitation to embark on therapy.

Treatment consisted of functional dental orthopedics to reposition the mandible and alleviate pressure in the temporomandibular joint next to the ear. This positional change allowed the normalization of function involving the ossicular chain, blood flow, muscular balance, neurologic impulse flow and lymphatic drainage. Within one week the ringing in the ears completely disappeared. The cause was definitely structural because the ringing returned within fifteen minutes after removing the orthopedic appliance. Twelve months of wearing the appliance caused structural changes that prevented the jaw from being displaced upward and backward. The second phase of therapy involved fabrication of a partial lower denture to support the new jaw height. Not only has Louise's ringing stopped, but also the sinus congestion, fatigue, ear stuffiness, neck stiffness, headaches, and joint noises have all resolved.

## VASCULAR – EAR CONNECTION

Since the blood vessels that supply the ear represent some of the smallest in the body, they are often the first to be narrowed by plaque. This internal corrosion consists of deposits of cholesterol, fats, calcium, heavy metal toxins, such as aluminum, cadmium, lead, guanidine (a toxic by-product of protein metabolism) and by-products of drug metabolism. As the circulatory system of the ear clogs, a progressive hearing loss develops. The circulatory system is also adversely affected by a deficiency of vitamin F (unsaturated fatty acids: linoleic, linolenic, and arachondonic). Natural fats are destroyed by the processing and refining of foods and the heating of oils during cooking. Vitamin F is essential for normal functioning of many organ systems and specifically is needed to push calcium into body tissues. Without adequate amounts of vitamin F, calcium is deposited in the lining of blood vessels, in body joints, and within the synovial joints between the middle ear bones causing a reduction in their mobility. Common ear problems that arise are tinnitus and conductive hearing loss.

From a functional dental aspect, the blood vessels to the ear branch off the internal maxillary artery whose beginning branch is opposite the neck of the mandibular condyle. Dental malocclusions will distort the condylar position; this distortion in turn, has the potential to disrupt blood flow to the ear. Whiplash injuries are another source for positional jaw distortions. Because of the muscular interrelationship among the neck, shoulder girdle, and mandible, the resulting spasms of neck muscles will force the lower jaw into a more retruded position. This also has the effect of disrupting normal muscle balance and cranial dura, bone and suture position, head posture, neurologic function, blood and lymphatic flow, and total body balance resulting in the gamut of physiologic aberrations. Physical traumas to the head or jaw may have similar influences including pelvic distortions resulting from dural and muscular interrelationships.

# DENTAL – PHYSIOLOGIC CONNECTION

## Case Study

Heather, a 7-year-old, was the youngest headache patient I had ever treated. Heather's mother had brought her daughter to my office for a routine dental examination. One look at the child's malocclusion prompted a whole series of inquiries. The mother seemed puzzled that a dentist should be asking questions regarding headaches, constipation, allergies, and other medical problems. After the initial shock wore off, the mother expressed an interest in her child's dental problem especially since Heather had been suffering from several major problems that later were revealed to be related to the malocclusion.

Prior to the family's moving to our area, Heather had been treated for five years by an allergist. This medical specialist had been injecting the child with serums in an attempt to alleviate the severe headaches, earaches, constipation, and general allergies. The mother told me that Heather would lie in bed and cry because the headaches were so severe. A major clue to the problem was the observation that the biting surfaces of her primary teeth had been severely worn flat. When questioned, the mother stated that her daughter would grind her teeth so loudly at night that it was noticeable from outside Heather's room.

Heather's dental problems of a decrease in jaw height and retrusion of her mandible started the fall of her physiologic dominoes. Because the bite was overclosed, the chewing muscles were not at their proper length. As the muscles shortened they went into spasm and strengthened (Davis' Law). In Heather's case, the temporalis muscle, which is a large fan shaped muscle located bilaterally over the temporal region, went into severe spasm. Since this muscle spans the temporoparietal suture, which connects the temporal and parietal bones by a long bevel joint, it caused a physical jamming. Squeezing the sutural area caused compression of the nerve endings which affected blood supply and resulted in severe headache pain. The grinding and clenching of the teeth was nature's reflex mechanism attempting to release the jammed suture. Grinding, clenching, and clamping the teeth together has the effect of causing the jaw-opening muscle, the external pterygoid, to go into spasm, which then refers pain into the middle ear.

A jaw imbalance will effectively place noxious stimuli into the nervous system and institute the triad effect that Dr. Selye spoke about in his General Adaptation Syndrome. The constant stress will cause the thymus and other lymphatic tissue to shrink, the adrenal glands to become hyperactive and the stomach to ulcerate. The lymphatic tissue is vital to the body's immune system and if hypoactive it will predispose the host to disease. The adrenal glands perform many functions, one of which is to maintain balance within the body when inflammatory agents like histamine are released. Ulceration of the stomach lining will permit undigested protein to enter the blood stream and initiate an allergic response. Poor digestion will also exacerbate an allergy problem by not breaking down the proteins into the simpler amino acid form. One of the effects of chronic sympathetic stimulation is the reduced motility of the intestines, which in turn causes constipation. An increase in waste evacuation time increases the level of body toxicity. If attempts are made with drug therapy to mask the symptoms of physiologic imbalances, then the body will be fighting a losing battle. True healing occurs when the cause of the problem is removed, allowing the body to heal itself.

The great French philosopher, Voltaire, appropriately summed up the body's healing capabilities when he stated, "The art of medicine is to amuse the patient while the body heals itself."

Although Heather presented various symptoms that at first appeared to be unrelated, there was a common denominator to her medical problems. That underlying factor was her dental malocclusion. The goal of therapy was to remove the structural imbalance as quickly as possible and allow the body to heal itself. Heather's bite discrepancy manifested a loss of jaw height accompanied by a retrusion of the mandible. Treatment involved use of a functional dental orthopedic appliance. The Bionator appliance used served to orthopedically reposition the jaw downward and forward and simultaneously allow the posterior permanent bicuspid teeth to erupt without interference from spastic chewing muscles, the tongue, or the cheeks. One week after the insertion of the corrective appliance, Heather's severe headaches, ear pain, and constipation were gone. Five months into treatment all her allergies disappeared. Completion of orthopedic treatment required two and one half years.

## Case Study 2

Ezra was 12 years old at the time his mother brought him to the office. The chief concern was the possibility of a cavity in a permanent molar tooth. Clinical evaluation established that no decay was present. However, Ezra presented a severe malocclusion which involved deficiencies in the vertical, horizontal, and saggital planes. A board-certified orthodontist recommended removing the first four bicuspid teeth to make space for the remaining crowded front teeth. Fortunately for the child the mother was reluctant to have any teeth extracted.

At the time of the initial visit, the mother was questioned about various symptoms that related to a malocclusion. The mother then proceeded to tell her tale of woe. Ezra was plagued with chronic severe headaches, severe allergies, and a hip joint that would always pop out during his participation in active sports. She presented a list of the various clinics, physicians, chiropractors and other health professionals she had sought to relieve Ezra's problems. Although some symptomatic relief was obtained, complete resolution never materialized. Treating symptoms with drugs and manipulating compensatory structural imbalances will only temporarily relieve the clinical symptoms. Therapy must focus on correcting the primary causative factor. In Ezra's case the keystone of the entire puzzle was the malocclusion.

The narrowed upper jaw physically restricted the lower jaw from coming forward. In addition, the "V" shaped maxillae created restrictions of cranial bone mobility and torqued the dural tube. The dural tension in turn placed a restriction on the sacrum. Since the sacrum sits between the two hip bones, they become dysfunctional and affect the hip joints and ultimately leg lengths. The temporomandibular joint (TMJ), like all the other joints of the body, possesses nerve endings which function to alert the brain of constant body positional changes and malfunctions. These receptors enable the body to limit joint motion as a reflex protective mechanism when one or more joints develops an abnormality. When traumatized, nature protects an injured joint by initiating spasms in those muscles that enable the joint to move. Because the body works in a reciprocal arrangement with other body parts, restrictions in the ranges of motion will occur to preserve the integrity of the whole system.

Ezra enjoyed soccer. However, every time he played his hip joint would go out. It was almost a ritual that after a game he would go to the chiropractor for an adjustment to correct the hip joint. The correction would hold only until the next game or other demanding physical activity. An interesting change took place about midway through dental orthopedic treatment. At the time, the upper jaw, which is composed of the two maxilla, had been widened by an orthopedic expansion appliance. The increased horizontal change in bone structure was adaquate enough to release the cranium and torquing on the dura allowing the sacrum to assume a more normal position. Ezra, his mother, and the chiropractor were all amazed that his hip joint did not misalign after several consecutive soccer games.

During the initial phase of treatment, Ezra's headaches disappeared. This was attributed to the repositioning of the lower jaw forward and an increased height. After orthopedic treatment to expand the bone structure, orthodontic therapy was used to align the teeth. Another fascinating aspect of the case materialized during the latter phase of treatment. The severe allergies that had previously plagued Ezra began to subside. All previous attempts to alleviate the allergy symptoms utilizing vitamin therapy and serum injections had failed. To date Ezra describes his allergy problem as only a minor nuisance.

The frightening aspect of this case and others similar to Ezra's is the "dental wisdom" possessed by many university orthodontic programs and their subsequent graduates. Conventional concepts focusing primarily on nonphysiologic, mechanical treatments are being presented to parents. In most instances the concerned parent wants a better aesthetic result. Although extraction of first bicuspid teeth is a necessary approach in a small percentage of cases, it has been used too frequently as an expedient method of correcting crowded teeth. If Ezra had been subjected to extraction of all four of his first bicuspid teeth, his problem may have been exacerbated. Ezra was already in trouble structurally and would have been made worse by conventional orthodontic techniques. Closing the extraction spaces by bringing his front six teeth backward would have jammed the lower jaw farther back and worsened the overbite. The cranium and cranial sutures would have become more restricted and the torquing of the dural tube would have increased. The added physical and neurologic stress to his system would have exacerbated the existing symptoms and created many more.

When a patient presents symptoms to the physician, it means that a state of dysfunction exists. The treating physician's primary objective should be to relieve the pain and suffering by removing the causative factors and to recommend any beneficial lifestyle changes. Frequently however, physicians as well as dentists concentrate on treating just the symptoms with mechanical appliances and drugs. When the symptoms resolve, we are led to believe that a "cure" has been established. In reality, eliminating the symptoms only forces the body to compensate over a prolonged period with potentially damaging consequences. For example, giving aspirin to suppress a fever only serves to mask the symptom. The fever is the body's own reflex mechanism to rid itself of toxic wastes. By suppressing a natural healing mechanism with drugs, the original toxins plus those added by the breakdown of drug products remain in the system longer and further stress the body. To prevent being treated symptomatically, the patient should question the doctor regarding the proposed dental treatment. Some thought-provoking questions are provided to stimulate the doctor/patient rapport:

1. Is my body deficient in any of the drugs that you are recommending to treat my symptoms?
2. What vitamins or natural substances can be used to treat my symptoms?
3. How important is my present diet in relation to my symptoms?
4. What natural healing alternatives are available?
5. Will osteopathic, chiropractic, or physical therapy treatments be of benefit in my TMJ therapy?
6. Is the recommended dental orthopedic appliance designed to treat the symptoms or effect a dental correction?
7. Will prolonged use (six months or more) of the dental orthopedic appliance depress my posterior teeth?

Many dental appliances presently being used will work well as a temporary measure. They are primarily designed to separate the teeth in an attempt to relax spastic muscles. Unfortunately, some patients discontinue dental treatment because of the false sense of being cured. They reason that since the symptoms have disappeared, they no longer have the problem. Dependence on the appliance often creates a heightened state of fear in which the patient believes he cannot exist without it, is afraid of damaging it, or even worse, of losing it. When the patient reaches this state of dependence there is a very good chance that the posterior molar and bicuspid teeth supporting the appliance have been depressed into the supporting bone. At this point the patient is worse off than before treatment was started.

8. Is the derangement in the temporomandibular joint caused by my collapsed bite or is it due to direct trauma or disease within the joint?

Often the symptoms of pain, clicking, swelling, etc., are localized in the joint itself. However, the actual source of the problem may be a loss of posterior tooth support, malocclusion, cervical distortions (misalignment of vertebrae and muscle spasms), pelvic rotations, or cranial bone misalignment. Some specialists may attempt surgery as a primary means of correcting the problem. I am not against surgery if documentation, e.g., by arthrogram (an x-ray that is taken after an opaque dye is injected into the TM joint to help confirm a torn ligament, anteriorly displaced joint disc or disc perforation) of joint derangement really exists. Even if true joint derangement is confirmed, the poor bite may have been the cause and may have to be corrected prior to surgery. Stability of the joint may require osteopathic and chiropractic manipulation as well as dental support. Surgery alone may create more problems since it does not correct the length of the chewing muscles, cranial, neck and pelvic areas.

9. Will I require orthodontic treatment utilizing full braces in connection with orthopedic therapy?

10. Will it be necessary to rebuild my bite with capping, partial, or full dentures at the completion of treatment?

*Warning: These questions may be detrimental to your doctor's ego.*

The information presented represents a level of knowledge on the leading edge of a new super speciality. Many of the clinical approaches have resulted from integrating osteopathic, chiropractic, physical therapy, and nutritional concepts. A physician must be open-minded enough and willing to dig laterally for the solutions. My experience with most universities and practicing physicians has been just the opposite. Some even have gone so far as to label such concepts as quackery. This I believe stems from ignorance, insecurity, and an unwillness to admit that maybe some of the conventional teachings are incorrect. This arrogant attitude is clearly seen in the statement, "... aerodynamically, bumble bees cannot fly." Obviously, bumble bees do fly but not so obvious is the fact that perhaps the accepted principles of aerodynamics are not yet wholly complete.

## THE TEN YEAR DENTAL EARACHE

Alice was referred to our dental practice by our hygientist. The patient's chief concern, at the initial visit, was to have her front teeth capped for cosmetic reasons. Dental evaluation revealed a collapsed bite and distorted lower jaw posture. As a teenager, she had lost several teeth and the remaining teeth had shifted into a convenience position. For a 45-year period, the patient's body had the awesome task of adapting to change. The altered dental complex had placed a heavy burden on the cervical vertebrae, musculature, and associated structures. The added dimension of time provided wear and tear, and a point was reached beyond which the body could no longer cope with the structural imbalance. When this overload prevailed, the symptoms appeared as warning signals.

While gathering information regarding past medical history, some major complaints surfaced. Alice had been suffering for a 10-year period with the problem of radiating right ear pain and numbness in the right cheek that had defied all medical attempts to diagnose or resolve. Interrelated and connected to the ear problem was a restricted cervical rotation to the left. Although Alice was skeptical about my interpretation of the dental-ear connection, she nevertheless agreed to proceed with a diagnostic appliance.

Therapy began with an orthopedic upper appliance that was designed to expand the maxillae. Four months of treatment brought about a miraculous change. Both the radiating ear pain and facial numbness completely disappeared. Another welcome surprise was the disappearance of the neck stiffness and rotational restriction. Alice remarked,"I didn't realize the extent of the cervical restriction until it vanished." The most noticeable change occurred while driving her car. Prior to treatment,"...it was always an effort to turn my head to see if traffic was clear. In order for me to effectively maneuver my head around I had to rotate my chest." Convinced of the efficacy of dental correction Alice agreed to continue with orthodontic treatment to properly align the teeth. A slight setback occurred when the orthodontic braces were removed. The ear pains and neck problems returned, however, not at the original intensity. The difficulty arose because of a lack of posterior vertical tooth support. Orthodontic techniques were incapable of forcing the molar and bicuspid teeth out sufficiently to provide the physiologic vertical support. The next phase of treatment focused on restoring all the upper teeth. By fabricating and applying fixed dental bridgework, the problem of an insufficient vertical support was overcome. As added insurance, a special micro-precision attachment was used between the two front caps. The purpose of this device was to permit the physical connection of the two front teeth and at the same time allow for normal micro–motion of the cranial bones. Once the dental bridgework was completed, Alice remained pain free and retained the flexibility of her neck.

## DIZZINESS AND MALOCCLUSION

Marie came to the office somewhat panicky and deeply concerned about dizziness and other seemingly unrelated symptoms. In the week preceding her office visit she had experienced a severe dizzy spell at work which completely incapacitated her. As a precautionary measure, she had been taken by ambulance to the emergency room at a nearby hospital. A neurological evaluation was negative and the attending neurologist recommended a dental evaluation for possible TMJ dysfunction. Prior to this emergency, Marie sought medical evaluation for complaints of facial numbness and tightness, chronic headaches on the back right side of the head, and ear, and lower back pain.

As is so often the case in patients with TMJ dysfunction, Marie presented a deep overbite and retruded lower jaw. The whole domino scenario with reciprocal structural changes came into play. The collapsed and retruded bite cause the cervical vertebrae to stack up straight like a military neck. The head goes into a forward head posture to reflexively open the airway for improved breathing. Muscle spasms result from the shortened posterior neck muscles while the anterior ones stretch and weaken. The structural impact of all these distortions is torquing of the dural tube which ultimately will have an influence on the cranial bones. Since each temporal bone houses an organ of balance and most likely each will be distorted in a slightly different plane, severe dizziness will result. Other factors such as stress, low blood sugar, hypoadrenia, decreased blood supply to the brain (caused by crimping of the vertebral artery as it passes through the distorted upper cervical vertebrae) and distortions of the head and neck can have major implications. Systemically the body experiences severe structural, physiologic and mental distress with an end result of chaos.

Overlaying Marie's structural distortions were a stressful job and poor eating habits. Applying the principles of the Physiologic Adaptive Range Concept, effort was made to remove as rapidly as possible those factors over which we had some degree of control. Cranial manipulation was performed to release jammed cranial sutures. Myofascial release techniques were employed to resolve the tissue contracture present in the cervical musculature. Marie was also instructed to eliminate, as much as possible, the basic nutritional stressors like caffeine, refined sugar, white bread, dairy products (because they have a tendency to clog up the lymphatic system) and saturated fats (margarine, butter and hydrogenated oils). Nutritional support in the form of natural B-complex vitamins, calcium, magnesium, trace minerals, and vitamin F (unsaturated fatty acids) were supplied. The pelvis was balanced by a non-invasive sacro occipital technic which utilizes padded wedges under each pelvic bone. The key disruptive dental factor was eliminated by supporting the patient's bite in an improved physiologic position. Cold helium neon laser therapy was directed to the master acupuncture, auricular (ear acupuncture points developed by the French physician Paul Nogier), TMJ and muscle trigger points. This approach goes beyond the conventional wisdom of Western medicine which focuses on treating the symptom. Eastern medicine, on the other hand, seeks out the root causes of the problem and corrects through the use of non-invasive methods such as nutrition and manipulative techniques. Removing the major distress factors will put the body back within a physiologic range, thus enabling it to continue to heal itself.

Within three weeks, Marie began experiencing relief. The dizziness along with the headaches, ear pain, facial numbness, muscle spasms, and lower back pain completely vanished. Treatment will continue with the use of a dental orthopedic appliance and orthodontics. Such therapy will require 2 - 3 years for completion.

## THE $18,000 HEADACHE

When Edna first came to my office, she was in severe pain and had contemplated suicide. The seemingly unrelated chief complaints of left ear pain, severe right upper and lower tooth pain, severe left facial pain, chronic neck and shoulder pain, lower back pain, and pains in both feet brought Edna to her peak of pain tolerance. Fate apparently was on Edna's side because the day she visited her family dentist to check out the tooth pain, he received my TMJ brochure in the morning mail. The dentist x-rayed the involved teeth but found no decay or abscessed teeth. He then referred Edna to my office for evaluation.

Edna's story of woe began in August of 1980 when she was treated by a podiatrist. The original complaint was pain in both feet. After a thorough examination of the localized areas of the pain, the podiatrist recommended surgery to reconstruct the bone to alleviate the pressure on the nerves and thus eliminate the pain. Following surgery, the patient was instructed to wear custom-designed shoe inserts. Within a week, Edna began experiencing lots of pain, first in her legs, then in her hips, and finally it settled in the lower back. Approximately two weeks following this episode, the pains subsided and her body entered the resistant stage of stress which required a myriad of structural and physiologic compensations.

Chaos began on March 5, 1981. Edna was suddenly struck with severe pains in the stomach, chest, and upper arms, and she began experiencing weakness in both legs. The family doctor immediately put Edna on the drug, Tagamet, for what first appeared to be an ulcer problem. To confirm his tentative diagnosis, an upper gastrointestinal test was performed. The results were negative. On March 18th, Edna was sent home from work because of severe chest pains and increased blood pressure. Her physician ordered a complete blood work-up and electrocardiogram and placed Edna in the hospital for four days for observation. On March 22nd, she was dismissed from the hospital and instructed to take eight extra strength Tylenol per day, Sorbitrate four times per day (used for angina attacks) and Nitrostat when needed for angina attacks. The extensive series of tests conducted by the hospital were all negative. These included stress test, SMA-25 blood work-up, gall bladder, liver, and pancreas studies. During April and May Edna's symptoms subsided again.

In June of 1981, Edna's symptoms exacerbated. The cervical pains worsened and the leg weakness became so severe she could hardly walk. A neurologist was consulted. X-rays of the involved areas revealed only a slight arthritic condition in the cervical area but proved negative regarding any structural abnormality or frank pathology. It was becoming apparent to everyone involved that Edna's situation was deteriorating.

In July of 1981, an osteopathic physician was consulted for possible relief of the severe pains in the back, jaw, ear and arms. The diagnosis was lumbosacral strain and osteopathic manipulation was provided. The manipulative techniques brought relief for the first time since the whole incident started. However, with the relief of the back pain came exacerbation of severe pain in upper and lower right tooth segments. Edna was now coming to the realization that she may have to live with this pain.

In October of 1981, The family dentist was consulted to evaluate the increased intensity of the pain as well as other facial areas that were being affected. Edna was now experiencing pains under the border of the right side of the jaw, bilateral pains behind the ears, right side facial pain and pain behind the right eye. Accompanying these symptoms was paresthesia which began affecting the right side of the face intermittently. All basic dental problems were ruled out.

In desperation, the patient went back to the podiatrist for an evaluation. His observations proved fruitless and he stated that he could find nothing wrong.

On November 3, 1981, Edna presented herself to me for evaluation. She was at her lowest point, suffering from frustration, depression, and hopelessness and was in severe facial pain. Because of Edna's obvious state of desperation, a dental orthopedic appliance was fabricated out of silicon putty. The patient was instructed to wear the appliance as much as possible. Another appointment was scheduled to continue the examination and try to solve the puzzle.

Edna returned for her next scheduled appointment. During the period of one week, 75 per cent of the facial pain had resolved. The patient was estatic but was made to understand that a cure was not at hand. The examination revealed some interesting findings. Although the bite appeared normal, x-rays of the temporomandibular joint showed the jaw joint to be displaced upward within the confines of the joint space. In addition, the cranium had jammed sutures and cranial bone distortions. Compounding the problem was the existence of an unstable, weak sacroiliac joint with hypermobile ligaments. Accompanying the structural imbalances were organ and nutritional problems. The prolonged stress to the entire system had caused the adrenal glands to be in hypofunction. There was a liver–gall bladder problem as evidenced by the patient's inability to handle fatty foods. There was an overconsumption of refined foods, too much protein, and a lack of minerals such as calcium, magnesium, zinc, etc. If one case ever had to be selected from my files as a model representing an all-encompassing dysfunction of the five major areas (cranial, dental, pelvic, physiologic and psychologic) Edna's would have to be the one.

With the assistance of Dr. Steven Lesse of Marlton, New Jersey we assisted Edna's body to heal itself over a period of a year. To help stabilize the jaw posture, an orthopedic appliance, a bionator, was used. Concomitantly, cranial adjustments were performed. In addition, Sacro-Occipital blocking techniques were used to re-establish stability to the sacroiliac. Dr. Lesse also corrected cervical and thoracic vertebrae distortions. The patient was put on an exercise program to be carried out at home. Diet modification was recommended and carried out with a high degree of compliance. Nutritional supplementation provided support for the adrenal glands, liver and gall bladder, weak ligaments, mineral deficiency and poor digestion. After about six months of treatment, Edna began to stabilize; however, adjustments to the sacroiliac would only hold for a period of several weeks and some of the symptoms would reappear. Out of frustration, I called my good friend Dr. Nelson DeCamp in Lakeland, Florida. After explaining our predicament, he suggested that foot levelers be fabricated to help stabilize the pelvis. This man's chiropractic genius solved the puzzle by providing the key factor that served to stabilize the entire structural frame.

In retrospect, Edna's scenario unfolded like a textbook case. The multitude of complaints definitely interrelated with the structural domino effect which occurred in her body. Edna's primary structural problems focused on a lowered vertical jaw position and a weakened sacroiliac joint. Prior to the appearance of foot pain, Edna's body was able to adapt to these structural imbalances. Interestingly, one of the first clinical signs of an unstable sacroiliac joint involves pains in the knees, ankles, and feet. What the podiatrist diagnosed as a local problem was in reality a major area of compensation. The invasive surgical procedure served only to upset the total body structure by traumatizing the area of compensation. The patient's problems progressively worsened. This resulted from other compensatory areas having to bear the burden of the original weakness plus the overlay of the disturbed balancing ability caused by surgery on the feet. Distortion of the spine and torquing of the dural tube forced the cranial bones to further compensate. Pressure on the fifth cranial nerve (trigeminal) which supplies the upper and lower teeth, gums, and jaw bone caused the previously unexplained pains. The seventh cranial nerve (facial) also became involved, thus accounting for the facial pain. The patient's body was in chaos and incapable of adapting. Only through a truly holistic approach utilizing the efforts of a well-trained SOT chiropractor, dental orthopedics, nutritional support, dietary changes, and the cooperation of the patient, was success achieved.

Edna has once again become a productive human being. She has been able to return to full-time employment and now leads a normal life. The irony of this case is the fact that the insurance companies paid $18,000 in workman's compensation, diagnostic tests, doctor, hospital, and drug bills but refused to pay the dental fee of $950.00 to get the patient well. To add insult to injury, the final physician's report for the workman's compensation board purposely deleted both the dental and chiropractic findings and therapeutic procedures. Incidences like this one certainly give one the impression that the establishment healers do not want to recognize nonconventional approaches to healing, especially when they are successful.

## TEN SETS OF DENTURES AND STILL NO RELIEF

You would think that after having ten sets of full upper and lower dentures a patient's problem would be solved. Marcelle's nightmare started 23 years ago when all her remaining upper teeth had to be removed because of gum disease. Six front teeth in the lower jaw were left and a partial denture was constructed. Within days after the dentures were inserted Marcelle began experiencing pains in both ears and in the head. Her medical merry-go-round had just begun. Specialists in many fields including neurology and ENT (ear, nose and throat) were consulted. All tests and clinical examinations were negative. As with many of these patients they are told they must live with the pain and accompanying symptoms.

Four years following the onset of the symptoms, Marcelle was still searching for relief. In desperation another dentist was sought for construction of a second set of dentures. At the time of the initial examination, this dentist felt the problem was due to lack of space between the back part of the upper and lower dentures. In an attempt to correct the problem, Marcelle was referred to an oral surgeon. The surgeon proceeded to remove "excess" bone and gum tissue to increase clearance between the dentures. The surgery created more room and the dentist went on to make the new dentures.

The second set of dentures brought no relief. Marcelle was still plagued by chronic ear and head pains. Through the years her situation continued to deteriorate. Marcelle's original symptoms now became overlayed with periodic general malaise, cloudy thinking, and neck and throat pains which worsened after eating and talking. The only source of relief was removing the dentures whenever possible. Marcelle went through at least eight more sets of dentures during the next 19 years. While the last two sets of dentures were being fabricated, she insisted that the bite be increased, but each time the dentist refused to comply.

In the end perseverance paid off. Marcelle got lucky and hit the jackpot. Fate directed her to a dentist who not only specialized in dentures but also was knowledgeable about the many symptoms associated with improper denture support. This prosthodontist referred her to my office for evaluation.

While Marcelle was telling her story of woe, it became obvious why she was experiencing such a wide variety of symptoms. In fact, it was the patient who actually provided the key information that enabled her problem to be solved. Examination revealed motion restrictions in the neck plus severe spasm of two muscles involved in opening the jaw. Treatment consisted of myofascial release techniques to release the tightness in the neck. The spasms of the jaw-opening muscles were resolved, and Marcelle's lower denture was relined to increase the denture height. The patient walked out of the office feeling immediate relief after suffering needlessly for more than 20 years.

At the follow up visit, Marcelle stated that her head, neck, and ear pains were gone and that she was more clear-headed and able to read the newspaper in the morning. Reading the newspaper is taken for granted by most people; however, Marcelle was unable to function adequately to accomplish this simple task. Another positive change was noticed by her husband, who commented on how her whole disposition had changed for the better. All this occurred within one week of correcting the denture height and eliminating the muscle spasms.

## "JAWLASH"

In the 1970s the term "jawlash" began appearing on dental reports as part of the sequelae of whiplash injuries. Because the jaw is attached to the skull and shoulder girdle through numerous muscle attachments, it easily becomes misaligned when the involved muscles go into spasm.

In a study conducted by the Preventive Dental Research Foundation, 500 whiplash injury cases were reviewed and considered "closed" after conventional treatment. The unfortunate victims, however, did not consider themselves cured, for they still suffered from a multitude of symptoms. According to the president of the research group, Dr. Harold Ravins of Los Angeles, the chief complaints included:

1. Pains of the head
2. Burning sensations of the forehead and scalp
3. Facial pains
4. Clicking, popping, or cracking sounds in the jaw
5. Buzzing, ringing, and roaring sounds in the ear
6. Stuffiness or itchy feeling in the ears
7. Balance problems
8. Difficulty in swallowing
9. Pain in the roof of the mouth
10. Blurred vision
11. Sensation of pressure around and behind the eyes
12. Sensitivity of the eyes to light
13. Reduction of arm and shoulder movement
14. Tingling sensations in the arms and fingers

Dr. Ravins and the other members of the Foundation traced these symptoms back to the violent, uncontrolled forces that had snapped the patients' heads around and misaligned their jaws.

The actual mechanism of whiplash involves a very complex, dynamic series of stretching, compressive and twisting forces dissipated throughout the skeletal structure and living soft tissue. A simplistic view portrays the event as a forward hyperflexion, and backward hyperextension with a corkscrew effect on the spine, sacrum, and pelvic complex. The sudden pulling and jerking motions created by the impact have the potential to cause ruptures and micro-tears within the muscle tissue. The microscopic changes within the muscle serve to exacerbate the pain. They include:

1. Decreased circulation of blood to the area
2. Decreased oxygen supply

3. Decreased ability of the lymphatic system to clear the traumatized area
4. Reduced nutrient supply
5. Increased metabolism of the involved tissue
6. Increased build-up of waste products
7. Increased muscle fatigue
8. Inflammation
9. Swelling

These changes account for the prolonged symptoms of muscle soreness and pain. The aftermath of the trauma also is characterized by latent secondary effects such as pressure on nerves and blood vessels from spastic muscles. Neurologic pressure will produce clinical symptoms of muscle weakness and tenderness, numbness, hypersensitivity, burning sensations, heaviness, paresthesia and shooting pains. Vascular pressure, on the other hand, will lead to decreased blood to an area, discoloration (such as in cyanosis), swelling and nutritional changes.

Whiplash injuries are not always the result of motor vehicle accidents but can result from falls, direct traumas to the skull, or moving forces applied to various parts of the body such as those which occur in contact sports. Whiplash should not be thought of as a typical syndrome, nor any particular injury but should be looked upon only as the mechanism of the injury. From a total structural perspective, other commom symptoms include:

1. Restriction of neck motion
2. Blackouts
3. Chronic fatigue
4. Heaviness of the head
5. Mental fogginess, lightheadedness, poor memory and inability to concentrate
6. Nausea and other gastrointestinal problems
7. Low back pains
8. Pain between the shoulder blades
9. Cold hands and feet, numbness of the arms, hands, feet and shoulders
10. Stress-related symptoms of extreme nervousness, palpatation, insomnia, excessive sweating, anxiety, depression, tremors, and pallor

Recent clinical experience indicates that as many as 80 per cent of whiplash injuries induced by rear-end motor vehicle collisions will also include associated TMJ trauma. These jaw joint problems do not necessarily appear immediately after the accident. In fact, some patients may not be plagued until months later. The primary trauma comes from the forces generated by the hyperextension phase. As the head is forced backward, the lower jaw is pulled forward and open. The TM joint ligaments and chewing muscles become overextended inducing micro-tearing within the tissue; then spasm and disc derangement occur within the temporomandibular joint.

# FOLLIES OF CONVENTIONAL WHIPLASH THERAPY

## Case Study 1

Pat was involved in a motor vehicle accident a little over one year ago. Like most whiplash victims she had no previous history of neck pains or headaches. However, she did have a malocclusion which predated the accident. Pat's dental problem involved an extremely deep overbite partly due to genetics and partly due to missing molar and bicuspid teeth. The improper bite was compounded by the backward tilt of the two upper front incisor teeth. The reversed inclination of these teeth physically restricted the lower jaw into a retruded position. The compensatory mechanisms caused the following changes: The normal 17 degree cervical vertebral curve was straightened; a forward head posture was induced; and a muscular strain was placed on the shoulder girdle and all involved musculature. Pat's body was able to adapt to these imbalances until the whiplash injury. The muscle spasms that resulted from the trauma overloaded an already compromised body.

The patient was subjected to all the conventional drug therapies which included muscle relaxers, anti-inflammatory drugs, and pain killers. In addition, all forms of physical therapies were tried: diathermy, ultrasound, cryotherapy, moist heat, and massage. Even osteopathic manipulation was used in an attempt to release cervical vertebrae distortions and muscle spasms. Out of desperation, the treating osteo-pathic physician brought the patient into the operating room and under general anesthesia attempted to release the severe cervical restrictions. The efforts were futile.

As a last resort, Pat was finally referred to my office. After fifteen months of symptomatic treatment, the original com-plaints were overlayed with chronic compensatory changes such as fatigue and depression. The chief complaints presented at the initial visit to my office were:

1. Chronic headaches (2 to 3 per week)
2. Extreme heaviness of the head
3. Chronic neck pains and spasms (Under physical stress the left side of the neck would balloon out and reach the size of a grapefruit)
4. Cracking of right and left TM joints when chewing and talking
5. Painful muscle on the right cheek area
6. Mental fogginess and forgetfulness
7. Deep seated ear pains
8. Periodic dizziness
9. Difficulty in opening the mouth

Examination of cranial function revealed a dis-harmony in the primary cranial rhythm (motion of the brain) and also in the secondary motion which was asynchronous with the normal diaphragmatic or breathing cycle. The cervical tissue contracture was severe, and rotational head movements were restricted and painful. The patient's diet included a high percentage of refined sugars and saturated fats, but lacked fiber, fresh complex carbohydrates, and minerals.

Treatment was aimed at first balancing the cranial rhythms by means of gentle cranial manipulation. Myofascial tech-niques were used to help release the long-standing cervical muscle spasms and fascial restrictions. The patient was instructed to avoid harmful refined foods and stimulating and depressant drugs like caffeine and alcohol. Nutritional sup-port was provided in the form of concentrated food supplements.

An all natural B-complex was given to help metabolize the excess lactic and pyruvic acid accumulation in the spastic muscles. Calcium, magnesium, and trace minerals helped restore muscle tone to a more normal relaxed state. Unsaturated fatty acids assisted in the diffusion of calcium into the muscle tissue. Because of the chronicity of the patient's problem and predominance of physical fatigue, the adrenal glands were supported with protomorphogens, substances that provide the building blocks for healing of the organ tissue and stimulate the hormones they produce.

Since the cervical area was dysfunctional from two sources (the dental malocclusion and the spasms brought on by the whiplash injury), support to the causative area (dental complex) would be necessary to resolve the symptom area (neck). First, resin bonding was placed on the biting surfaces of the remaining posterior teeth. This served to prevent the jaw from overclosing and disrupting the integrity of the temporomandibular joint. It also established a more normal physiologic length for the chewing muscles as well as those of the neck and helped correct the compensatory forward head posture. Further support was provided with the use of an orthopedic appliance. Although the appliance was removable, the design enabled the lower jaw to be held in a stable position in much the same way as a cast holds broken bones. The bionator orthopedic appliance functioned also to help restore, as best as possible, the normal curve of the cervical vertebrae. Dental support was the keystone to the structural imbalance. Within three visits, mobility in Pat's neck started to improve. To assist in the release of muscle spasms, soft helium laser was directed to the meridian acupuncture points in the web spaces of the hand, ear acupuncture points, specific TMJ acupuncture points and the Ah Shi (muscle trigger) points.

Since physiologic dentistry was implemented, the patient has had a dramatic turn around of symptoms. The extreme heaviness of her head has virtually disappeared. Ear pains have vanished. The headaches have been tremendously reduced in frequency and intensity. The ballooning of the left neck flexor muscle has been reduced to the size of a golf ball instead of a grapefruit. Pat's mental clarity has improved, and she now sees light at the end of the tunnel.

This case, as well as the others, points up what the author has been emphasizing throughout this book–find the causes and treat them. Unfortunately for the American people, Western medicine focuses its attention on treating the symptoms and tries to control them with drug therapy. The other frightening aspect of the traditional medical delivery system is their interpretation of a holistic approach. Basically it espouses the philosophy of shipping the patient from one specialist to another until each runs out of his/ her bag of tricks or drugs. A true holistic approach entails treating the total patient with as non-invasive an approach as possible. Manipulative techniques, good nutrition, nutritional support, psychological counseling, dental support when necessary, cranial therapy and acupuncture all of which must be integrated with the sophisticated techniques of modern medicine. Each has its place, and the deciding factor in utilizing one approach over another should not be based on the practitioner's economic status or inflated ego but the welfare of the patient.

**Case Study 2**

Dolores was first seen in my office on an emergency basis. The immediate problem was severe cervical pain and bilateral jaw pain. At this visit treatment was rendered to help alleviate the patient's pain. Cold, helium–neon laser was directed to the associated acupuncture, auricular, TMJ and muscle trigger points. Myofascial release techniques were used to free up the cervical muscle tensions caused by spasms. The patient was then asked to return for an extended visit for a thorough evaluation. Dolores returned in a week and presented the following chief complaints:

1. Constant pain at the lower left angle of the jaw
2. Chronic headaches
3. Chronic neck pains
4. Ringing sounds, primarily in the left ear
5. Limited range of neck motion

As is so often the case with whiplash injuries, the cranial rhythms become disrupted. The combination of muscle spasms, distorted motion of the original trauma spread along the dural tube, and distortions of the pelvis, sacrum, vertebrae and cranium all have the potential to cause an irregular motion of the primary and secondary rhythms. This motion distortion in turn impedes nerve impulse transmission, and normal flow of cerebrospinal fluid into the brain, down the spinal cord, and out along the spinal nerves. The potential for motor and sensory problems plus disruption of normal physiology anywhere in the body is great.

Dolores exhibited an irregular primary and secondary cranial rhythm. Complicating this already disturbed motion was the existence of extensive jamming of cranial sutures. In addition, numerous cranial bones had restricted ranges of motion. In essence, the skull's motion was diminished while the cranial bones were being pulled inward by the dural tube which was torqued from the trauma of the accident.

A pre-existing dental malocclusion placed the patient into a structurally compromised state of adaptation. Lacking proper dental support because of several missing molar and bicuspid teeth helped reduce the normal curve of the cervical vertebrae. Dolores' body was constantly fighting to maintain some semblance of balance without any trauma. The whiplash injury tipped the scales to such a degree that the body could not recuperate on its own. It is for this reason alone that such patients are bounced around from one specialist to another without responding to conventional therapy. Proper occlusion or bite relationship is one of the major factors in maintaining proper body balance (among the skull, spine, sacrum and pelvis). If this vital link is broken, structural integrity is lost and the patient may be labeled a hypochondriac, malingerer, neurotic, or other convenient classification. Even worse than being labeled, some of these unfortunate souls are subjected to exploratory surgery when all else fails.

Dolores also had distortion of the lower lumbar vertebrae and pelvis. Of interest in patients with this distortion is the consistent finding of a painful first rib head (located on the back side bilateral to the spine about the level of the shoulder). When the sacroiliac goes out, increased motion occurs at the point where the rib attaches to the spine and usually results in pain. Furthermore, a pelvis distorted by rotation with one ilium posteriorly rotated (short leg side) and the other in anteriorly rotated (long leg side) will cause one leg to be functionally shorter than the other. If by chance the quadratus lumborum muscle (which extends from the eleventh and twelfth ribs and attaches to the five lumbar vertebrae and superior crest of the ilium) is in spasm it also has the potential of creating a functional short leg.

To assist the patient in achieving structural balance, the pelvic complex was corrected with the use of Dr. DeJarnette's padded wedges which allow the body's own weight to make the change. Cranial manipulation was performed to release the jammed sutures. Next, dental support was provided. Myofascial release techniques were then used to release the cervical area. Soft laser was directed to the associated acupuncture points and muscle trigger points.

Dolores was placed on a vitamin regimen for muscle spasms and counseled nutritionally. To support structural correction, the patient was referred for full body massage therapy and chiropractic care. Within a period of two months, the headaches and cervical pains were greatly reduced.

One major variable that played a continuing role in perpetuating the patient's muscle tension problem was psychological distress. The emotional aspect was related to personal family problems. Often this information surfaces only after the doctor has gained the patient's confidence. Nevertheless, the patient must attempt to lessen the impact of the emotional upsets in order to achieve a higher degree of treatment success. In Dolores' case a plateau has been reached in therapy and progress will now depend on the patient's efforts.

## Case Study 3

Jo Anne is a 44-year-old homemaker who had suffered with chronic headaches for the past ten years. Her medical history seemed at first uneventful. However, approximately two years prior to her visiting our office, Jo Anne had completed orthodontic treatment for a retruded lower jaw and deep overbite. The treatment plan required the removal of two upper first bicuspid teeth to provide space to retract the remaining six front teeth. Although the bilateral spaces were adequately closed and the teeth aligned, the lower jaw became physically restricted in the retruded position. Also the deep overbite was not sufficiently corrected. The malpositioned lower jaw set in motion the entire adaptive body posture. The previous headaches worsened as a result of the structural change.

About a year after completion of orthodontic therapy, Jo Anne was involved in a motor vehicle accident. The whiplash injury not only exacerbated the pre-existing headaches but also established severe neck pains and constant toothaches. The conventional treatment package of a soft neck collar, Valium, and physical therapy did nothing to relieve the pains.

While at a social gathering, Jo Anne mentioned to my secretary that she had been suffering for a number of months with headaches, neck pain, and toothaches. Knowing the potential involvement of the jaw, neck, and headaches in whiplash injuries, my secretary recommended that Jo Ann set up an appointment for an evaluation.

The examination revealed the fact that the jaw joints were posteriorly displaced and were putting pressure against the ear canals. When kinesiologic muscle testing techniques were used, they verified that the over-closed and retruded lower jaw posture was aggravating the spastic neck muscles. The combined effect of the perpetuated malocclusion and whiplash injury was torquing of the dural tube. The original headache was caused by a collapsed bite which was due to incomplete eruption of the natural teeth. The additional induced traumas served to heighten the distortion. To effectively alter the strained musculature and lost cervical curve, a removable orthopedic appliance (bionator) was inserted. By the third month, the symptoms were greatly alleviated. Continued wearing of the appliance for another six months virtually erased the complaints.

## Case Study 4

Shelly was referred to our office by her physical therapists. In 1981, she was involved in a motor vehicle accident in which she was struck from the rear. In the emergency room she was provided with Valium and a soft collar. Next came traditional physical therapy which included ultrasound, Hydroculator packs and electrical stimulation to the sore muscles. These treatments brought minimal relief.

When Shelly presented herself for evaluation her main complaints were:

1. Left ear pains especially upon awakening
2. Pain and pressure behind the left eye
3. Shooting pains starting from the left shoulder and progressing to the back of the head
4. Constant dry mouth
5. Limited opening of the mouth
6. Constant tightness of the chewing muscles

Examination of the dental structures revealed that her jaw was retruded as a result of the spastic neck muscles and straightening of the cervical vertebrae. The jaw joints were compressing against her ear canals, especially on the left side. All the chewing muscles were in spasm and her jaw opening was limited to 35 millimeters (normal 40 to 65 millimeters). The right and left jaw joints had audible clicks. The left joint also produced crepitation (grinding noise similar to that produced when walking on pebbles). The chiropractor's report stated that Shelly's cervical spine had a right rotational fixation of the first two cervical vertebrae, and palpation of her cervical and thoracic spine revealed areas of exquisite tenderness throughout with numerous trigger zones. The blood chemistry showed low readings for the red blood cells, hemoglobin, and sugar levels. The white blood cell count was high which indicated an infection.

The clinical composite, which included muscle pain, tightness, and limited ranges of motion, job-related stress, and inability to sleep and eat properly, quickly caused Shelly's physical and mental status to deteriorate. To get the patient back into a better physiologic adaptive range, treatment focused on nutritional support, chiropractic manipulation, and dental orthopedic support.

Nutritionally, the patient was given B-complex vitamins (help to break up the metabolic waste products within the muscles), vitamin C (great detoxifier, supports the adrenal glands, aids healing of tissue, and in high doses acts as an antihistamine), an adrenal concentrate (to support adrenal function), Hemadyne (a product which supports the production of red blood cells), digestive aids (hydrochloric acid and pancreatic enzymes), calcium (for tissue integrity and spastic muscles) and vitamin B-6 and magnesium to act as a natural diuretic (helps reduce swelling due to fluid build up). The patient responded well to the combined treatment. By the sixth week most of the symptoms were gone. The dental orthopedic appliance was discontinued since the muscle tightness and limited jaw opening had resolved. The irony of the whole case was that although the physical therapists were delighted with Shelly's rapid recovery, they stopped sending referrals. Their reason was based on the fact that they were getting their referrals from an orthopedic surgeon who did not hold chiropractors in high esteem.


# FACTS CONCERNING
# TISSUE INJURY AND REPAIR


Tissue injury associated with whiplash creates a period of crisis for the body. The physiologic demands needed to protect the organism and repair the damage are increased manyfold. Under normal circumstances, the 100 trillion cells of the body are breaking down at the rate of 24 billion per day. In each cell there are between 300 and 800 power plants called mitochondria. Within each mitochondrion (in the liver) there are approximately 5,000 respiratory units, while each mito-chondrion in the heart contains as many as 20,000 respiratory units. The 70,000 miles of blood vessels that transport the body's fluids contain 30 trillion red blood cells. The normal, healthy individual produces 15 million red blood cells per second to replace the same number that are destroyed. That turnover represents 900 million red blood cells per hour. Cognizant of this awesome complexity, one must give serious concern to the quality of food ingested to support this magnificent machine and the potentially harmful effects of drug therapy.

In order for a cell or group of cells to be replaced, the following conditions must exist:

1. A constant blood supply for the delivery of oxygen, and nutrients for the removal of metabolic wastes and carbon dioxide

2. A constant nerve supply with nerve impulses which activate and regulate cellular function as well as regulate the blood supply

3. An adequate supply of:
   a. a full spectrum of naturally occurring vitamins
   b. a full spectrum of minerals
   c. a full spectrum of trace mineral activators
   d. a full spectrum of enzymes

4. Proper lymphatic drainage of tissue spaces and required white blood cells to assist in local defense of an invader and for tissue repair

No matter what the cause of the tissue injury, the body must utilize several biochemical and physiologic activities to replace or repair the damaged tissue.

The first stage in tissue injury is the process of inflammation. Defined by *Dorland's Illustrated Medical Dictionary*, 25th Edition, inflammation is "a localized protective response elicited by injury or destruction of tissue, which serves to destroy, dilute, or wall off... both the injurious agent and the injured tissue." In the acute form, inflammation is characterized by the classical signs of pain, heat, redness, and swelling.

Another respected source of medical information is the *Textbook of Medical Physiology* by Arthur Guyton, M.D. In the 6th Edition published in 1981, Guyton states on pages 70-73: "Inflammation is a complex of sequential changes in the tissues in response to injury. When tissue injury occurs...large quantities of histamine, bradykinin, serotonin, and other substances are liberated by the damaged tissue into the surrounding fluids." The released histamine functions to increase blood flow into the injured area causing a state of "brawny edema" (thickening of inflammation) or congestion in the spaces surrounding the injured cells. Dr. Guyton continues, "It is clear that one of the first results of inflammation is to 'wall off' the area of injury from the remaining tissues." And,"...the intensity of the inflammatory process is usually proportional to the degree of tissue injury."

Based on these two sources of information, it would be a safe assumption that inflammation is a necessary and essential protective response in the healing mechanism. Why then would a physician prescribe an antihistamine drug to reduce the swelling of a post-whiplash injury? It would seem logical that such a drug would interfere with the first stage of healing. Even ingestion of large amounts of ascorbic acid will have a disruptive effect. Increased quantities of ascorbic acid pharmacologically act as a neutralizer of histamine. The accumulation of histamine functions to activate the second stage of the healing process.

The second phase of healing involves the state of hyperemia. As the volume of blood to the area of trauma increases, the traumatized area becomes reddened and warm. The elevated temperature is also part of the healing process. Dr. O.P.J. Falk, assistant professor at St. Louis University School of Medicine, said, "Fever represents an effort by the body to accelerate the metabolic process ... any attempt to control fever artifically, is defeating nature's purpose." The biochemistry of inflammation requires the presence of the fever as an essential part of the repair process. This truth was substantiated by a double-blind study conducted by Dr. Falk. He found that flu patients who were given aspirin were disabled twice as long and had 3 1/2 times more complications than those patients who were given sugar pills.

Exercise, sexual activity, and eating will cause a normal increase in body temperature, while a drop will occur during an individual's deepest sleep. In conditions of cold weather and in the early morning, body temperature may reach a low of 96° F. At the other extreme, Guyton cautions of the possibility of cellular damage when the temperature exceeds 106° to 108° F.

In the July 1980 issue of the *Journal of Clinical Therapeutics,* it was stated that most authorities regard temporatures below 106° F. as harmless and those over 108° F. as potentially harmful.

A University of Colorado pediatrician, Dr. Barton D. Schmitt, conducted a study which revealed that most people are overly concerned about fever. Dr. Schmitt feels that these fears are unjustified, since serious complications are rarely produced by fevers (Am J Dis Child 134: 176-181, 1980).

Robert S. Mendelsohn, M.D., author of *Confessions of a Medical Heretic*, stated emphatically that, "Temperature taking is virtually useless because there are innocuous diseases that carry very high fevers. Roseola, for example, is a common disease of infancy, absolutely harmless; yet it frequently carries a temperature of 104° or 105° F. On the other hand, there are life-threatening diseases, such as tuberculosis, meningitis and others, that carry no fever at all, or even a subnormal temperature."

Rothenburg, a physiologist, and Dr. Kluger, at the University of Michigan Medical School concluded, that taking drugs to reduce fever may well impair the body's own protective defense facilities. Aspirin may combat pain, but indiscriminate use to reduce fever may be a serious human error.

When the body exhibits heat and fever, it indicates that the first line of defense is functioning. The acutely ill patient who lacks a fever is the one to be concerned about.

The third stage witnesses the influx of white blood cells (WBC) which have the capability of digesting foreign bodies. These white blood cells begin the task of cleaning up the area of damaged tissue. If not interfered with, the process of inflammation can continue until completed. However, administration of antibiotics and/or steroids actually hinder this phase. From the book *The Influence of Antibiotics on the Host-Parasite Relationship,* comes the realization that antibiotics impair the body's immune system. These antimicrobial drugs will prevent the migration of white blood cells to the area of inflammation, and will impede the ability of the scavenger white blood cells to engulf and destroy foreign bodies.

Dr. Widmann of Johns Hopkins and many others have revealed that the majority of antibiotics are antimetabolites and actually function to inhibit cell membrane synthesis. Laboratory tests show that antibiotics work differently in the test tube than in the body. Antibiotics will kill microorganisms in the glass petri dish by weakening their cell walls. Within the patient, however, the real effect of antibiotics is to block enzymatic reactions of cellular biochemistry needed for tissue repair or replacement. In summing up the effectiveness of antibiotics, Dr. Richard Murray was accurate when he stated, "The administration of antibiotics during the course of an inflammatory process is analogous to putting out a fire by dousing it with gasoline."

In the final analysis, use of drugs will only relieve the symptoms. If an antihistamine is taken to prevent swelling, then the first stage of inflammation is disrupted and tissue repair will be delayed. Prescribing an antipyretic (aspirin or similar drug) will stop the hyperemia (increase of blood volume) with its accompanying heat and fever, but again the repair process will be retarded. Administering an antibiotic or steroid will provide symptomatic relief but without any tissue repair. Unfortunately most patients treated thusly will be delighted because their symptoms have been controlled. In the long run, however, the patient's body will pay the price.

# Part IV

# Nutritional Aspects
# Of Headaches And Disease

# "THY FOOD SHALL BE THY MEDICINE"

The age of specialization has produced health practitioners who deliver medical services in much the same way that fast food chains provide their patrons with goods and services. Professional training is so specialized that practitioners never really get a total concept of how the body interrelates physiologically, structurally and nutritionally.

The typical American diet is high in protein, refined sugars, and saturated fats and low in natural fiber, whole grains, fresh fruits and vegetables, nuts and seeds, high quality protein, and unsaturated oils. In reality, Americans are functioning on "low-octane" fuel, and are developing widespread degenerative diseases at a young age. The solution to our health problems was provided by Hippocrates over 2500 years ago when he stated, "Thy food shall be thy medicine, thy medicine shall be thy food." Nutritional deficiencies when coupled with environmental pollutants, stress of daily living, and structural imbalances set up individuals for their medical problems.

## GENETIC OR DIETARY DETERIORATION ?

The old saying that America is the land of plenty aptly describes our nation's health status -- plenty of degenerative diseases. Approximately one-half of our population is afflicted and suffering from such maladies as cancer, heart disease, stroke, hypertension, diabetes, arteriosclerosis, cirrhosis of the liver, obesity, mental illness, cataracts, arthritis, multiple sclerosis, tooth decay, gum disease, and loss of teeth. Of the top ten leading causes of death in the United States, six (heart disease, cancer, stroke, diabetes, cirrhosis, and arteriosclerosis) are degenerative diseases. Over one million Americans will die each year of heart attacks and strokes. Diabetics now number in excess of 10 million. Over 5 million Americans are victims of arthritis. Approximately 33 million people are considered to have succumbed to mental illness. The number of children classified as hyperactive, retarded, and schizophrenic is steadily on the rise. As bad as this may appear, drug consumption is even more alarming. Americans consume an estimated 37 million pounds of aspirin each year. We lead the world in chronic headache sufferers with an estimated 45 million. We also swallow 1 1/2 million pounds of tranquilizers and 836,000 pounds of barbiturates. Americans shell out over one-half billion dollars a year on Valium and other so-called headache remedies. Degenerative disease is not due solely to the fact that we are living longer, because today more than ever, our young people suffer from these same chronic illnesses. We are touted as having the highest standard of living among the nations of the world but our people are truly the sickest to walk this globe.

At no point in the history of civilization has man been subjected to such cruel and unusual punishment in the form of processed foods. Man's body has been pushed to its physiologic limits in attempting to adapt to adulterated food. In its wake, the ravages of degenerative diseases have appeared.

Based on the United States Department of Agriculture surveys from 1910-1976, American consumption of wheat fell 45 per cent, corn 85 per cent, rye 78 per cent, barley 66 percent, buckwheat 98 per cent, beans and legumes 46 per cent, fresh vegetables 23 per cent, and fresh fruit 33 per cent. During this same period intake of beef increased 72 per cent, poultry 194 per cent, cheese 322 per cent, canned vegetables 320 per cent, frozen vegetables 1650 per cent, processed fruit 556 per cent, ice cream 852 per cent, yogurt 300 per cent, corn syrup 761 per cent, and soft drinks 2,638 per cent. To further add insult to injury, the intake of chemical additives and preservatives since 1940 has risen by 995 per cent.

At the turn of the century, man's demise was due primarily to infectious diseases such as pneumonia, tuberculosis and influenza. At present, too many Americans are so heavily burdened with degenerative diseases that their energies have been diverted from pursuing the good life. For some, seeking symptomatic relief via allopathic (traditional) medicine has become a full-time endeavor. The vast majority, however, seem to be sputtering through life like a car whose motor pings from the effects of low-octane fuel. The chosen few who return to consuming food of the highest quality will reap the good feelings that so many others in our society attempt to derive from mood-altering drugs. The afflicting scourge will continue its devastation until man changes his diet back to a balance that is in harmony with nature. Only when we resume the consumption of whole grains, fresh vegetables, freshly prepared soups, beans, and sea vegetables, and quality protein will the disease statistics begin to abate.

Since there are no time outs in this great game of life, we must live each day with quality by embarking upon it with a good positive attitude, physical health, high-octane nutritional foods, and pursuit of our goals.

## ONE LIFE TO LIVE *

You've only got one life to live
So live it in peace, live it in truth, live it in love

And then you live each day
Like it's your last one
You take control of your emotions
All your doubts and fears

And just as the world, and all it's sadness
And replace joy for those salty, bitter tears

'Cause you've got one life to live
So live it in peace, live it in truth, live it in love

And you greet every day
with a little love in your heart
You go and do all the things you desire
All the things you dream of
Because today is the beginning of a brand new life
You have to fail sometimes
In order for you to succeed

You got one life to live
So live it in peace, live it in truth, live it in love

If you're feelin' down and out let's sing

If you're sad I'll make you laugh

And if you become puffed up with too much pride
Remember that everything, everything must pass

You got one life to live
So live it in peace, live it in truth, live it in love

You've got one life to live
So give it your all

Give it a lot
Give it your best shot

\* Copyright Mighty Three Music
Blackwood Music Inc., Kenny Gamble and Leon Huff

These words may sound familiar. They make up a song
that was popularized by Lou Rawls. Its lyrics make up a creed
to live by. One of its writers, Kenneth Gamble, had this to say
about *One Life to Live:* "Life—the most precious gift of all. The
chance to experience physical things and spirited things at
the same time. The Creator of life is greater than life. There
is no greater treasure than a life of awareness —being aware
of the purpose of life. That purpose is to glorify and exalt the
Creator; to be humble, to be caretakers of the physical
condition. We are blessed every day we wake up. To destroy
life is a sin; to destroy the earth is a sin.

"Just as every snowflake has a different design, so do the
patterns of life. There has never been another you, or another
me, on this planet before. We've got one life to live...so let's
live it in peace, truth and [nutritional] harmony."

## THERE ARE NO MAGIC BULLETS AGAINST DISEASE

Present day state-of-the-art medicine has led the public to
believe that the medical practitioner alone has the magic
bullets against disease. Unfortunately these magic bullets are
falling short of their targets. As a nation we have dropped
from seventh in the world to sixteenth in the prevention of
infant mortality; in female life expectancy we have dropped
from sixth to eighth; in male life expectancy, we have dropped
from tenth to twenty-fourth. We are failing despite spending

more than 75 billion dollars on medical care. That is more money being spent than by any other country on the face of this globe. Emmanuel Cheraskin, M.D. summed up our plight when he made the statement, "The plethora of such pronouncements makes it now abundantly clear that health is the fastest growing failing business in these United States."

The well-documented work of Drs. Weston A. Price and Francis C. Pottenger [available from Price-Pottenger Nutrition Foundation, 5871 El Cajon Blvd., San Diego, CA 92115] brings to light the effects of cooked protein on the degenerative process. Their study was conducted on two groups of cats. One group was fed a diet of cooked protein and pasteurized milk while the other group ate only raw protein and raw certified milk. After three generations of cats, the clinical findings were observed to mirror man's present nutritional plight. The group of cats fed the cooked protein exhibited during their life span many of the degenerative diseases of man. They suffered from arthritis, cirrhosis of the liver, colitis, ulcers, gum disease, loss of hair, heart problems, clogged arteries, cancer, cataracts, constipation, tooth loss, and other diseases. The toxins produced, (a result of the breakdown of cooked protein) in these cats were so poisonous that even noxious weeds would not grow where they defecated. The second generation of cats from those fed cooked protein exhibited malformation of the upper jaw, and bone deformities; some were stillborn, while the remaining cats suffered many ills and died prematurely. The frightening aspect of this experiment was that there was no third generation of offspring from these cats.

On the other hand, the group of cats raised on the raw food enjoyed a healthy normal life. They reproduced healthy offspring who lived a normal life expectancy and who went on to produce a healthy third generation. Review of the degenerative disease statistics in this country will lead one to believe that the status of health in present day Americans parallels the second generation of the first group of cats.

The body's inherent ability to heal itself is tremendous. To support this innate power, one must combine knowledge, a positive attitude, quality food, exercise, and manipulative osteopathic or chiropractic care. The information in this section will provide insight into healing the body. By eating unprocessed foods the body will gradually detoxify itself and help reduce potential sources of headaches and other symptoms. It should always be remembered that "the road to health is through your kitchen, not the pharmacy."

## QUALITY OF FOOD

When discussing nutrition, we are in essence dealing with only three principal groups: proteins, carbohydrates, and fats. Establishing a diet that is right for you will require a basic understanding of each of these food sources plus some nutritional principles to follow.

# PROTEINS

Proteins are probably the most controversial of all nutrients in the field of nutrition. Whether a high or low protein diet is the most beneficial, or whether animal protein is superior to the vegetable form, or which protein is complete or incomplete seem to be the areas usually debated. Through a better understanding of the nature of the beast, you will be able to make your own final judgment.

Proteins are probably the most complex of all the known biological substances. They are the only sources of nitrogen complexes necessary to build protoplasm which constitutes the physical basis of all living cells. Proteins provide the chemical structure for the body's enzymes, antibodies, hormones, blood plasma, lymphatic fluid, and other substances. There are simple proteins like albumins and globulins and complex ones represented by nucleoproteins which are the basis of ribonucleic acid (RNA) and deoxyribonucleic acid (DNA). Other complex proteins are phosphoprotein, which is the principal protein of milk and egg yolk. Additional examples are chromoproteins (hemoglobin), lipoproteins (in brain tissue), metalloprotein (iron-containing protein) and others.

All proteins contain carbon, hydrogen, oxygen, and nitrogen; most of them also contain sulfur, and some contain phosphoprus. Elements such as iron, iodine, copper, manganese and zinc are also present but their presence depends on the nature of the protein. The basic building blocks of protein are the amino acids which become available to the body during digestion of protein. There are an estimated 435 trillion different combinations that can result from the 22 amino acid units which comprise the thousands of formed proteins. The body can produce all but eight of the 22 amino acids (L-Tryptophan, L-Phenylalanine, L-Lysine, L-Threonine, L-Valine, L-Methionine, L-Leucine and L-Isoleucine). These eight are referred to as the *essential amino acids* and must be supplied by the diet. In addition, all the essential amino acids must be present simultaneously and in proper ratios in order for the body to produce proteins.

# DENATURING AND COAGULATION OF PROTEINS

Denaturing of protein refers to the rearrangement of the amino acids that occurs within the protein molecule when the protein is subjected to heat, acid, alkali, or other physical forces. On the other hand, if their solubility is lessened, the proteins are considered to be coagulated. The protein of an egg, for example, is coagulated and denatured when it is fried or hard-boiled. Similarily, when milk is pasteurized, its protein becomes denatured and the destroyed enzymes (phosphatase) prevent the utilization of calcium by the body.

An experiment conducted on newborn twin calves produced a result which strongly suggests that long established "scientific" dogma should be questioned. From the very first day, both calves were fed their mother's milk but one calf's portion was pasteurized. At the end of 60 days, the calf fed the pateurized milk died.

Meats, poultry, and fish undergo the same denaturing process when cooked. It is estimated that 80 per cent of the protein is destroyed by the act of cooking. When protein foods are cooked, 6 amino acids are inactivated. Five of these are essential and non-synthesizable by the body. Reheating these foods will serve to reduce what little nutritional value is left. Although not yet documented, use of microwave cooking has the potential to be more detrimental to health than conventional gas or electric cooking. Because microwaves are high energy waves they serve as more efficient means of protein destruction.

Most people consider hamburger as a convenience food and a source of nutritional protein. In reality, it is one of the more toxic decayed forms of ingested substances. As soon as the animal is slaughtered, the carcass begins to deteriorate. This decay process is slowed down by freezing; however, the formation of ice crystals within the tissues causes tearing and rupturing of cells which then liberate enzymes and other substances that hasten spoilage. The time factor must also be taken into consideration. Weeks may elapse from the time the animal was killed, shipped to meat packing plants, and redistributed to local markets, before it reaches your dinner table. The additional act of grinding the meat to create hamburger will release more enzymes and cause further tissue degeneration. Ingesting this toxic waste produces a major source of body odor while putting a strain on the organs of detoxification (liver, kidneys, colon, and skin), and the body's immune system, and provides a potential source of toxic headaches.

To derive the maximum nutritional value from protein, it should be cooked only minimally. Those individuals who have acquired a taste for sashimi, the Japanese delicacy of raw fish, are really obtaining one of the highest qualities of protein. Those concerned about the problem of parasites from eating raw or rare protein foods can greatly reduce the chance of this by taking a nutritional supplement called Zymex II (available from Standard Process Laboratories, 2023 West Wisconsin Ave., P.O.Box 652, Milwaukee, Wisconsin 53201; tel.# [414] 933-2100). As a proteolytic enzyme (capable of breaking down protein), this product is an excellent aid in the digestion of parasites.

## PROTEIN DIGESTION

Of the three principle food groups, proteins are the most difficult for the body to digest and utilize. Protein is handled in the stomach and small intestine. The chemical process by which proteins are digested is called hydrolysis. During hydrolysis there are a series of intermediary components with the end product being amino acids. Essential to this process is hydrochloric acid and a proteolytic enzyme–pepsin. The hydrochloric acid sets the chemical stage for activity while the pepsin helps break up the proteins into simpler amino acids.

As gastric emptying occurs, protein digestion is carried on by excreted pancreatic enzymes and intestinal secretions. The amino acids are rapidly absorbed through the intestinal wall into the systemic circulation for transport to the liver for detoxification and then to needed sites throughout the body. Consuming a diet high in refined foods requires less hydrochloric acid for digestion, and therefore the body produces less. As production of this acid diminishes, the body's ability to handle proteins becomes a problem. Exacerbating this situation is the intake of sugars along with proteins at the same meal. The sugars disrupt the digestive process setting the stage for improper breakdown of protein in the body. Partially digested protein causes fermentation and toxic waste build-up which leads to a multitude of symptoms: acid indigestion, stomach bloating, sour taste, putrified breath odor, foul-smelling bowels, itchy rectum, toxic headache, stomach ulcers, abdominal pain, diarrhea, colitis, increase of arthritic pains, fatigue, and others. Increasing age also brings about a reduction of hydrochloric acid production. Both factors result in a diminished quantity of available protein to the body. As protein deficiency ensues, the aging process progresses more rapidly.

## PROTEIN REQUIREMENT

Ten to 15 per cent of the daily caloric intake should be provided by quality protein. From a standpoint of maintaining health, a daily consumption in the range of 30 grams (equal to 1 ounce or 2 tablespoons) to 70 grams (equal to 2.5 ounces or 5 tablespoons) of an unaltered protein (minimally cooked) will be satisfactory for both males and females. Needs vary according to daily physical activity, age, and climatic conditions. Living in a colder climate will necessitate a higher protein consumption than someone residing in a tropical zone. As a general guide, a more exact figure can be calculated using the ratio of 1 gram (.04 ounces) of protein daily for each kilogram (2.2 pounds) of body weight. Since youngsters are in a rapid growth period they may require 2 grams (.07 ounces) per 2.2 pounds per day. Elderly people are usually in a state of negative nitrogen balance and will also require 2 grams (.07 ounces) of protein per kilogram (2.2 pounds) of body weight.

Research has established the fact that approximately 30 grams (1.06 ounces) of body protein are metabolized and used for daily body maintenance. This loss must be replaced by a new source of quality protein for daily energy and tissue replacement. Protein reserves can be maintained if the daily intake is 50-70 grams (1.75 to 2.45 ounces). An important point to keep in mind is that unaltered, complete protein is needed. However, individuals who are primarily vegetarian may be ingesting only partial proteins and may require an increase of complementary protein. A complementary protein is a protein that supplies the amino acids missing in another partial protein, thus making the combination more complete. As an example, brown rice is high in the amino acids Methionine and Cysteine but lacks Lysine. The Japanese food, tofu (soybean product), is high in its Lysine content. Combining brown rice and tofu at the same meal will provide a protein source that is approximately 92 per cent complete in all the amino acids.

The process of combining proteins was discovered long before the existence of the National Academy of Sciences, Food and Nutrition Board. Looking back in history, all traditional societies used protein combinations as the basis of their diets. The Asians combined soy foods with rice, wheat, millet, or barley. Middle Easterners consumed recipes which included bulgur wheat with chickpeas, or pita bread felafel with hummos (combination of whole wheat, chickpeas and sesame seeds). The Latin Americans were noted for their corn tortillas with beans or combination of beans and rice. The following general categories are offered as a guide for combining proteins:

Whole grains                 +    Legumes
  (millet, oats,                     (peas, beans,
  brown rice, buckwheat, etc.)       lentils)

Seeds and nuts               +    Legumes
  (sesame, pumpkin
  & almonds, chestnuts, etc.)

Whole grains                 +    Milk products
                                     (preferably raw
                                     certified)

Ideally people should eat only when hungry. This results in smaller meals throughout the day. The big advantage is that complementary proteins eaten within a few hours of one another would still be available for protein combining. In addition, less stress would be placed on the body's digestive and detoxification systems. For a more in-depth study of complementary proteins and their nutritional value, you are urged to read *Diet for a Small Planet* by Frances Moore Lappé.

Because of the widespread use of drugs in the beef and poultry business, consumers are urged to choose organically raised livestock. The antibiotics and steroid drugs ingested by eating contaminated protein will prove detrimental to health. As the quality of our food continues to decline, our immune systems become less able to deal with the common everyday variety of bacteria and viruses and even less capable of handling the more resistant strains.

From an everyday practical standpoint, one can obtain a high quality source of protein from eggs, seafood and complementary plant proteins. Following Benjamin Franklin's philosophy of "everything in moderation" would aptly apply to adding small amounts of a quality animal protein like turkey or fish to vegetarian delights.

## PROTEIN EXCESS

Research indicates that most Americans consume twice the recommended quantities of protein per day. Today's typical diet provides twice the recommended daily allowance of 5 ounces per day for a 154 pound male and 4 ounces per day for a 128 pound female. The average healthy individual can tolerate such excesses for only so long before nutritional side effects start appearing. These side effects manifest themselves in the form of vitamin and mineral deficiencies. A daily protein excess of 70 grams (2.5 ounces) of protein above the recommended allowance, coupled with 60 per cent refined carbohydrates and saturated fats (typical American diet) will lead to vitamin B-6, B-3, calcium, and magnesium deficiencies.

The University of Wisconsin's Department of Nutritional Sciences conducted a study on young men. The study revealed that significant levels of calcium were present in the urine when these men consumed a high protein diet. Low and medium protein consumption, however, caused no loss of calcium. It was the opinion of the researchers that a state of osteoporosis (porous, brittle bone due to demineralization) would occur as a result of excess dietary protein over a period of a decade.

Fast food restaurants have changed the eating habits of Americans and have contributed their share of the daily protein excesses (sales in excess of 55 billion hamburgers). The significance of lower levels of calcium and related mineral depletion is seen in the increased state of hyper-irritability among the general public. Decreased calcium levels allow muscles to go into spasm more easily, set the stage for tension headaches, provide the source for itchy skin during the winter months, fever blisters and cold sores during the summer, unexplained low grade fevers, and cramping of calf muscles and toes during the middle of the night. Further compounding the problem is the addition of carbonated sugar drinks. They have the effect of further reducing the blood serum calcium level. From an overall health standpoint, the average American is being set up, via numerous degenerative diseases, for pain and suffering with a greatly shortened life expectancy.

Presented in the lists that follow are symptoms of vitamin and mineral deficiency frequently caused by excess protein consumption.

### SYMPTOMS of VITAMIN B-6 DEFICIENCY

- Loss of hair
- Water retention during pregnancy
- Numbness and cramps in arms and legs
- Slow learning
- Temporary paralysis of a limb
- Increase in urination
- Muscle weakness
- Depression
- Cracks around the mouth and eyes
- Visual disturbances
- Neuritis
- Arthritis
- Heart disorders involving nerves
- Irritability
- Dermatitis

## SYMPTOMS of VITAMIN B-3 DEFICIENCY

- Muscular weakness
- General fatigue
- Loss of appetite
- Small ulcers
- Recurring headaches
- Nausea
- Insomnia
- Strain
- Deep depression
- Indigestion
- Various skin eruptions
- Bad breath
- Irritability
- Canker sores
- Tender gums
- Vomiting
- Tension

## SYMPTOMS of CALCIUM DEFICIENCY

- Nervousness (one of the first signs)
- Muscle twitching
- Muscle cramps, numbness, and tingling in arms and legs
- Heart palpatations
- Slow pulse rate
- Excessive irritability of nerves and muscles
- Osteoporosis
- Bone malformation
- Joint pains
- Insomnia
- Impaired growth

## SYMPTOMS of MAGNESIUM DEFICIENCY

- Coronary heart disease
- Blood clot formations in heart and brain
- Calcium deposits in kidney, blood
  vessels and heart
- Apprehensiveness
- Tremors
- Disorientation
- Muscle twitching
- Confusion

Excess protein is metabolized to produce energy in the same way that carbohydrates or fats are converted to calories. Once digested, amino acids are highly reactive and reorganize rapidly within the cell to form new protein. Newly formed excess protein is stored primarily in the liver, kidneys and intestinal lining. When protein consumption surpasses an optimum point, that is, amino acid and energy requirements have been met, the protein is converted into fat by the liver and stored within its cells. As the protein reserve site overloads, toxic products empty into the bloodstream. The metabolic wastes establish an acidic condition within the cells, bloodstream, and extracellular fluids, which are normally alkaline. Maintenance of an acidic environment will lower the resistance of the immune system, produce clinical symptoms of fatigue, headaches, and chest pain and will ultimately lead to degenerative diseases such as cancer, arteriosclerosis, cataracts, mental illness, and others.

An interesting case in point, is the decline of the incidence of cancer in Holland following the food shortages during World War II. A Dutch epidemiologist, Dr. F. de Waard, correlated the cancer decline (35 per cent to 60 per cent), which occurred in Holland between 1942 and 1946, to the food shortages. During the German occupation, most of the protein sources—cheeses, butter, milk, eggs, and meat, were requisitioned. The Dutch people were forced to survive on their home-grown vegetables, bread and other staples. Following the war, the routine protein sources were again available and the cancer rates returned to their original prewar levels.

Below are listed many of the effects of excessive protein consumption:

- Disruption of healthy intestinal bacteria
- Increased occurrence of diarrhea
- Distortion of the acid-base balance of body chemistry
- Liver function impairment
- Indigestion
- Increased quantities of uric acid, urea and toxic purines (cause depression)
- Increased fat in bloodstream (reduces available oxygen levels to organs, tissues, and cells)
- Hardening of the arteries
- Pyorrhea
- Arthritis
- Osteoporosis

- Premature aging
- Deficiencies of vitamin B-3, B-6, calcium, and magnesium
- Ammonia production (demonstrated to be highly carcinogenic)
- Depletion of pancreatic enzymes, depression of function of pancreas and interference with insulin production
- Increased nitrogen production (hazardous with any type of kidney problem)

International research has shown that the highest life expectancies (90–100 plus years), occur in those countries where protein consumption is low. Countries having diets high in protein correspondingly have the lowest life expectancies. Of all the industrialized countries in the world, the United States has the highest protein intake for adult males and ranks 21 in life expectancy. This poor showing is believed by many nutritional authorities to be the result of our high protein diets.

# CARBOHYDRATES

The body's chief source of energy is derived from carbohydrates. Structurally, carbohydrates are composed of organic compounds including carbon, hydrogen, and oxygen and are represented as sugars, starches, and cellulose in the foods we eat. Carbohydrates exist in three basic forms: the simplest, *monosaccharides,* of which glucose is the most important; the second form, *disaccharides,* are composed of two monosaccharide molecules and represented by sucrose (cane sugar), lactose (milk sugar), and maltose. The most complex group, the *polysaccharides* (glycogen, starch, and cellulose), are made up of enormous molecules of monosaccharides. Polysaccharides are obtained by eating natural complex carbohydrates (whole grains, fresh fruits and vegetables) and offer the added bonuses of minerals, enzymes, vitamins, and fiber. In comparison to proteins and fats, carbohydrates are the most easily digested and burn 100 per cent clean when releasing their energy.

Consumption of complex carbohydrates will provide the body with the most efficient source of energy. Eating whole grains such as brown rice, oats, rye, millet, buckwheat, and raw or lightly steamed fresh vegetables will produce a slow constant supply (estimated at two calories per minute) of glucose into the bloodstream. This occurs as a result of many digestive processes. Polysaccharides must first be broken down into simpler sugars and finally into monosaccharides before they can be absorbed. In contrast, monosaccharides and disaccharides are rapidly absorbed through the intestinal wall appreciably raising the blood sugar level. As an example, intake of four ounces of glucose will be absorbed within fifteen minutes whereas the same quantity of fructose (complex sugar contained in tupelo honey) requires about four hours. Once in the bloodstream, glucose becomes an efficent fuel. Being highly soluble, it can be transported anywhere in the body and utilized directly by body tissues. Excess amounts of glucose will be stored by the liver, muscles and other tissues in the form of a complex starch, glycogen. Upon demand, the liver and other tissues are capable of converting the glycogen reserves back into glucose.

When the immediate energy needs of the body are met and the limited storage depots are filled, excess glucose is converted into fatty acids and stored in the form of triglycerides. Although the body has a limited capacity to store carbohydrates it has an unlimited capacity to store fat. The conversion of glucose to triglycerides depends to a large degree on the quantity of insulin available. In cases of hyperinsulinism, insulin production is high and glucose is easily transformed into storage fat. A double crisis now evolves. First, the excess fat will infiltrate and surround organs decreasing their ability to function. Second, the high insulin production quickly lowers the blood sugar levels to a point where the body begins craving sugar. Even though the individual is physically full, the blood sugar demands have not been met.

The typical American diet, which is high in refined carbohydrate foods (white bread, pastas, donuts, candy, cakes, dried cereals, etc.) has the potential to oversensitize the beta cells of the pancreas forcing it to produce large quantities of insulin. The end result is an erratic blood sugar level which sends the individual on an emotional roller coaster ride and sets the stage for disease. Since the simple sugars are quickly absorbed, an overabundance of glucose occurs within the cells. This results in an imbalance of oxygen and causes incomplete combustion of glucose and production of organic acids (lactic, pyroracemic, butyric, and acetic). The cellular environment is now in a condition of acidosis compounding an already acid condition caused by the consumption of excess protein. When coupled with the acidic intra- and extracellular fluids, metabolic toxins will hasten degenerative diseases such as arthritis, cataracts, gum disease, diabetes, and cancer.

Daily carbohydrate consumption should comprise 50 to 75 per cent of the bulk of our diet. However, the exception to this would be for those individuals who live in colder climates. Since a colder environment requires the body to produce more heat, protein and fat intakes will have to be increased to meet the individual's needs.

Selection of complex carbohydrate foods should be based on several important factors. Only those foods that grow within your locality or similar type climate should be consumed. One just has to view the eating habits of animals to see this universal principle in action. Another universal principle is based on the ancient oriental philosophy of yin (expansive) and yang (contractive). Eating tropical fruits (yin) during the winter (yin condition) months is out of balance if you reside in Nebraska, Vermont, or other geographically cold areas. It is just as inconsistent for a Floridian to consume daily portions of beef, chicken, buckwheat, millet, or wheat (yang foods), while living in a warm (yang) climate.

Another serious consideration is the elimination of all vegetables or fruits that have been canned or frozen. The processes of pasteurization, freezing, and the latest "technological breakthrough," food irradiation, all have the effect of destroying whatever little nutritional value is left in the food. A concerted effort should be made to purchase organically grown fresh fruits and vegetables. Large commercial farms have depleted the soils by improper crop rotation and a lack of organic fertilizers, and they have contaminated our food supply with the use of pesticides and synthetic fertilizers. Finally, choice should also be based on the acid- or alkaline-forming properties of the food.

# TOXIC EFFECTS OF SUGAR

The major concerns of the patient suffering from whiplash type injuries are twofold: (1) to reduce the intake of toxic, processed foods and (2) to increase natural healthy foods which enhance tissue repair.

One of the biggest sources of toxicity comes from the intake of refined sugar. In 1982, the world population consumed over 92 million metric tons of sugar. Americans ingest sugar at the rate of 8 tablespoons every 24 hours. Sugar sources include processed foods and soft drinks which supply approximately 45 pounds of corn sugar per person swallowed each year while the sugar bowl accounts for an additional 77 pounds per person.

As a refined carbohydrate, sugar is devoid of vitamins, minerals, essential fats, and proteins. It supplies the body with little more than calories but has a damaging effect on the body. Since the refining process of sugar strips away the potassium, vitamins and trace minerals, the body becomes depleted as it must provide these nutrients for proper combustion. This noxious substance, sugar, has a direct effect on the health of the intestinal track by destroying the natural bacteria flora. These normal bacterial inhabitants are responsible for producing the B-complex vitamins, vitamin K, and glutamic acid. By forming lactic acid, their presence protects the intestine from the formation of bacteria of decay and disease. Once breakdown begins, the normal healthy Bacillus acidophilus, Bacterium coli and others transform into toxin-forming organisms. Their poisons are reabsorbed into the bloodstream and cause such symptoms as headaches, fatigue, nausea, colitis, fowl-smelling stools, bad breath, bladder infections, cracks in the corner of the mouth, constipation, burning tongue, bruising, nose bleeds, pruritis ani (itchy rectum), yeast infections, and others. These problems are also caused by antibiotic and steroid therapy since both drugs will destroy the normal bacterial flora.

As far back as 1948, Harold Lee Snow, M.D. documented the effect of refined sugars on the body's blood chemistry. For a period of 6 days after the ingestion of 4 ounces of candy, Dr. Snow graphed the blood serum levels of calcium and phosphorous. His findings showed that during the first six hours, the usable serum calcium dropped from a level of 78 per cent to 54 per cent. It wasn't until the fourth day that it returned to a level of 72 per cent and two additional days were needed to reach the original level of 78 per cent. Likewise, the serum phosphorous level decreased from 3.5 mg/dl to 3.1 mg/dl and required 5 1/2 days to return to normal. This information has more significance than most physicians and patients realize. Calcium, for example, is present in every cell of the body and plays an important role in the health of that cell. In addition, calcium is contained in the blood serum and helps maintain the acid-base balance of the body, is essential in the clotting mechanism, transmission of nerve impulses, and the contraction of muscle fibers, and prevents muscle cramping, helps prevent convulsions, maintains heart rhythm, is important in cell division, organ function, prevention of osteoporosis, anxiety, muscle pains, conjunctivitis, sunburn, sinusitis and helps to counteract heavy metal toxicity and radioactivity.

Phosphorus, like calcium, is also present in every cell of the body. The body's use of phosphorus is closely interrelated to its use of calcium and a constant ratio of 2 1/2 parts calcium to one part phosphorus must be maintained for optimum health. Phosphorus is necessary for the assimilation of fats, protein, carbohydrates and digestion of vitamin B-3 (niacin) and B-2 (riboflavin). Disrupting the calcium/phosphorus ratio will have disastrous effects on the body. According to Dr. Melvin E. Page, researcher and author of *Degeneration and Regeneration,* calcium/phosphorus imbalances will bring about such degenerative diseases as arthritis, pyorrhea, tooth decay, muscle weakness and others.

Dr. Snow summarized his testing with the following statements: (1) Refined sugar reacts like a drug not a food; (2) Sugar is obviously the cause of many diseases of childhood and infancy; (3) Sugar is addictive like alcohol; (4) Refined sugar is responsible for vitamin and mineral deficiencies; (5) Its use results in tooth decay, diabetes, indigestion, intestinal gas, skin diseases, anemia, obesity, respiratory membrane weakness, arthritis, tuberculosis, cancer, high blood pressure, fatigue, and (6) refined sugar is extremely difficult to avoid since it is added to most packaged, canned, and processed food.

As a general rule, all people must avoid the intake of refined sugar, especially those patients who are suffering the ills of whiplash trauma and/or any existing malady. Research by Emanuel Cheraskin, M.D. has documented sugar's effect on the immune system. Dr. Cheraskin's work showed that consuming even small amounts of refined sugar will effectively lower the white blood cells for a period of time. The body's white blood cells represent the defensive system that attacks and destroys foreign bodies, such as bacteria and viruses, that enter the blood stream. Essentially, one's overall resistance is lowered and susceptibility to infections increased as a result of sugar consumption.

Emotional stress will not only influence the entire body but will also compound the effects of sugar on the availability of calcium. Anxiety, fatigue, and nervous tension will produce the metabolic waste lactic acid. Lactic acid, in turn, will combine with the stored calcium in the muscle tissue. In order for muscle contraction to occur, calcium must be available to activate a specific enzyme. The accumulation of waste products within the muscle perpetuates the spasms, which prevents nutrients, oxygen, and blood from gaining access, places pressure on nerves, and slows lymphatic drainage. The end result is muscle tension, spasms and delayed healing.

With the use of the electron microscope, scientists have discovered that each cell in the central nervous system has a shell of some calcium compound within its cell wall. As the integrity of the cell wall is disrupted, the cell becomes irritable. When the calcium shell thins out, the nervous impulses become dissipated causing faulty motor and sensory activity. When such functional disturbances are coupled with diets high in refined foods, problems usually worsen and recovery is prolonged.

The brain differs from all other organs in the body in that it is nourished solely by sugar (glucose). Researchers Fabrykant and Pacella have shown that changes in the blood levels of sugar and calcium are accompanied by definite changes in the electrical activity of the brain. The brain also is more sensitive to changes in the level of sugar than any organ in the entire body. The ingestion of refined sugars will produce rapid high quantities of sugar which enter the bloodstream only to be counteracted by an increased production of insulin.

This scenario of sugar highs and lows creates an emotional rollercoaster ride for its victim. It becomes very obvious that a junk food diet, which is lacking in many essential nutrients, will have a major impact on the functioning of the brain and may cause many behavioral dysfunctional abnormalities.

## CHAOTIC EFFECTS OF HYPOGLYCEMIA

One of the most devastating maladies affecting Americans today is functional hypoglycemia. According to the United States Department of Agriculture, one person in every ten is adversely affected by sugar. Functional hypoglycemia involves a low blood sugar level which is not adequate to support the normal function of the nervous system and brain. Those afflicted will exhibit an unbelievable variety of symptoms:

1. Nervousness
2. Irritability
3. Exhaustion
4. Syncope (fainting, dizziness, cold sweats, feelings of weakness)
5. Depression
6. Vertigo
7. Drowsiness
8. Headaches
9. Digestive problems
10. Forgetfulness
11. Insomnia
12. Anxieties
13. Mental fogginess
14. Tachycardia (rapid heart beat)
15. Muscle pains
16. Numbness
17. Indecisiveness
18. Unprovoked crying spells

A general guide to establishing a true diagnosis of hypoglycemia must satisfy the three criteria of Whipple's Triad:

1. Many of the above symptoms must be present during a hypoglycemic attack.

2. A serum glucose test should be performed while the above symptoms are present; an immediate blood glucose level of less than 50 mg./dl must be recorded.

3. The ingestion of glucose will result in dramatic relief of symptoms.

True hypoglycemia is caused by pancreatic beta cell tumors, severe liver disease, pituitary or adrenal insufficiency, hypothyroidism, or excess alcohol consumption which prevents the formation of glucose. If the symptoms are primarily acute and occur infrequently, the disorder constitutes a functional, reactive hypoglycemia rather than a true hypoglycemia. The individual who is a functional hypoglycemic is the one who usually is wrecked by the ingestion of refined sugar. These people are the victims of vitamin B-complex deficiency which prevents the body from properly metabolizing the sugar. It is extremely interesting to note the symptoms of a B-complex deficiency as presented by Thomas Spies, M.D. and others:

1. Muscular weakness
2. Lassitude
3. Irritability
4. Depression
5. Memory loss
6. Headaches
7. Nervousness
8. Tachycardia
9. Anxiety
10. Apprehension
11. Morbid fears
12. Mental confusion

13. Rage
14. Hostility
15. Hypochondria
16. Noise sensitivity
17. Constant fear of impending doom

In reality, many people are being misdiagnosed and improperly treated. The principal objective in treatment of hypoglycemia is to remove the offending substances from the diet (refined carbohydrates such as candy, cakes, donuts, ice cream, white breads, sodas, etc.) and replace them with quality complex carbohydrates, proteins and fats. Diets such as the one proposed by the late Nathan Pritikin or the macrobiotic diet or any other eating concept that espouses consumption of natural whole grains, fresh vegetables, fruits, nuts, beans, and unprocessed, unsaturated fats will assist the body in maintaining an even blood sugar level. Excessive high and low blood sugar levels are avoided because complex carbohydrates metabolize more slowly and release a more constant supply of calories. If willing to accept responsibility for the nutritional aspect of therapy, the patient can become actively involved in the healing process and greatly increase the chances for success.

## ACID–ALKALINE BALANCE

Acid- and alkaline-forming elements are properties of all natural foods. The predominant inorganic matter is the principal factor that determines whether a food will produce an acid or alkaline residue. The acid-forming elements include sulfur, phosphorous, chlorine, and iodine. The alkaline-forming elements are sodium, potassium, calcium, magnesium, and iron. Although a food such as grapefruit may be acidic, its organic acids will be reduced to carbon dioxide and water. When metabolism is completed, the inorganic alkaline elements remain and neutralize the acids.

Paradoxically, acid foods will reduce body acids. On the other hand, animal protein is high in the sulfur-bearing amino acids and phosphorous, and most whole grains are high in phosphorous. Digestion of these foods will leave sulfuric and phosphoric acid, and therefore they are classified as acid-forming foods. The typical American diet, with its excess animal protein and refined carbohydrates, provides large quantities of acid forming foods. Consuming a daily regime of such foodstuffs has the potential of establishing an acid blood and extracellular environment. Clinically, the beginning stages will be observed as tiredness, loss of mental sharpness, and lowered resistance (frequent colds). As the fluid environment becomes more acidic, the symptoms will worsen and manifest as generalized pains such as headaches, chest pain, stomachaches, etc. For more information on this subject, read *Acid and Alkaline* by Herman Aikara (published by the George Ohsawa Macrobiotic Foundation, 1544 Oak Street, Oroville, California 95965).

From a practical nutritional approach, it is safe to consume a diet that is 60–80 per cent alkaline and 40–20 per cent acid. For convenience, an acid–alkaline chart is provided. Focusing on the selection of the proper complex carbohydrate foods will totally eliminate the need to count calories. Eating quality complex carbohydrates will provide a sense of well being and fullness without the bloating that accompanies ingestion of refined foods. Those making this change may experience intestinal distress (for weeks or months) in the form of increased gas formation. Past abuses of eating highly refined foods reduce the body's need to produce large amounts of hydrochloric acid and also help destroy the natural, healthy bacteria that live in the lower intestine. These bacteria are needed to break down the complex carbohydrates. To alleviate this problem it is recommended that a digestive aid, betaine hydrochloride, be taken with each meal. Until the stomach adjusts to the increased fiber and complex carbohydrates, two tablets may be necessary with meals. Such products are readily available at your local health food store. Additional help in relieving flatulence will come more quickly by restoring the normal, healthy bacteria. This can be accomplished by taking lactobacillus acidophilus, which is also readily available in health food stores. The ingestion of this supplement will convert carbohydrates to lactic acid in the gastrointestinal tract and make it easier to digest proteins, absorb calcium and iron, and assist in the detoxification of the body.

# ALKALINE FRUITS

Apples and apple cider
Apricots
Avocados
Bananas
  (ripened, speckled only)
Berries
Cactus
Cantaloupe
Carob (pod only)
Cranberries (slightly acid)
Cherries
Currants
Dates
Figs
Grapes
Grapefruit
Guavas
Kumquats
Lemons, ripe
Limes
Loquats
Mangoes
Melons
Nectarines
Olives, sundried
Oranges
Papayas
Passion fruit
Peaches
Pears
Persimmons
Pineapple, ripe and fresh
Plums (slightly acid)
Pomegranates
Prunes and juice (slightly acid)
Raisins
Tangerines
Tomatoes

# ACID FRUITS

Bananas, green-tipped
Cranberries
Fruits, glazed with raw sugar
Fruits, sulfur-dried
Jellies, canned or preserved with sugar
Olives, pickled green

# ALKALINE VEGETABLES

Artichokes
Asparagus, ripe
Bamboo shoots
Beans, green, lima,
or sprouts
Beets and tops
Broccoli
Cabbage, red and white
Carrots
Celery
Cauliflower
Chard
Chicory
Chives
Collards
Cucumber

Dandelion greens
Dill
Dulse (sea lettuce)
Eggplant
Endive
Escarole
Garlic
Horseradish, fresh
Kale
Kohlrabi
Leeks
Legumes (except peanuts
and lentils)
Lettuce
Mushrooms (slightly acid)
Okra
Onions
Parsley

Parsnips
Peppers, green and red
Potatoes (all varieties)
Pumpkin
Radishes
Rhubarb (oxalic acid forms
an insoluable calcium
salt)
Rutabaga
Sauerkraut
Sorrel
Soy beans (slightly acid)
Spinach (oxalic acid)
Squash
Taro, baked
Turnips and tops
Water Chestnuts
Watercress

## ACID VEGETABLES

Artichokes
Asparagus tips, white
Beans, dried
Beans, garbanzo

Brussels sprouts
Lentils
Rhubarb

## ALKALINE DAIRY

Acidophilus (natural bacteria
found in dairy products)
Buttermilk

Raw milk (human)
Whey
Yogurt

## ACID DAIRY

Butter
Cheeses
Cow's milk (boiled, cooked, pasteurized,
malted, dried, or canned)
Custards
Ice cream and ices (due to high refined sugar content)

# ACID PROTEIN FOODS

Gelatin (from animal protein sources)
Gravies
Red meats, fowl and fish
Seafood

# ACID CEREALS

Barley
Buckwheat
Breads, all types
Cakes
Corn, cornmeal, cornflakes, and hominy grits
Crackers
Flour products
Doughnuts
Dumplings
Grapenuts
Noodles (Macaroni and spaghetti)
Oatmeal
Pies and pastry
Rice
Rye-krisp

# MISCELLANEOUS ALKALINE SUBSTANCES

Agar (a white gelatin derived from a species of seaweed)
Alfalfa products
Ginger, unsweetened, dried
Honey, raw tupelo (absorbed more slowly than most honey and can be tolerated by most diabetics)
Kelp (can be used as a seasoning or condiment)
Teas, unsweetened
Alfalfa
Clover
Mint
Oat
Oriental
Sage
Strawberry
Yeast cakes

# MISCELLANEOUS ACID SUBSTANCES

Alcoholic beverages
Candy and other confectionery
Cocoa and chocolate
Coffee
Condiments (curry, pepper, salt, spices, etc,.)
Drugs
Eggs (especially the whites)
Ginger, preserved
Jell-O (contains 95% white sugar)
Flavorings
Food Preservatives:
Benzoate
Brine salt
Sulfur
Vinegar
Smoked foods
Marmalades
Mayonnaise
Sago (starch)
Sodas (loaded with sugars and phosphoric acid to increase
Tapioca (starch)
Tobacco (juice, snuff, smoking)

## ALKALINE NUTS

Almonds
Chestnuts, roasted
Coconut, fresh

## ACID NUTS

Nuts, all others (increase in acidity with roasting)
Coconut, dried
Peanuts

With respect to intestinal health and headaches, the body
benefits tremendously from a diet high in complex carbohydrates. By providing the intestinal tract with roughage in the
form of cellulose, the muscular tone of the intestinal wall is

maintained while the transit time of toxic wastes is shortened. By preventing constipation, the liver, kidney, and skin (largest excretory gland in the body) are spared the awesome task of removing the noxious wastes. In addition, the normal bacterial flora is preserved, which in turn produces the B-complex vitamins, vitamin K, and glutamic acid (essential for brain function) and enables the normal flora (acidophilus yeast) to convert the carbohydrates to lactic acid. The lactic acid will promote the growth of other healthy bacteria and will block the growth of toxin producing organisms. Taking bakers' yeast or brewers' yeast should be avoided since they will convert the carbohydrates into alcohol and carbon dioxide (cause of bloating) rather than into lactic acid.

Also blocked by lactic acid is the formation of guanidine, which is one of the most alkaline and toxic products in the body. This substance has been implicated as a contributing factor in toxic headaches, arthritis, hypertension, convulsions, muscular dystrophy, and epilepsy. Guanidine has the potential to cause calcium deposits in arthritic joints, muscle pain, arteriosclerosis, and is a specific calcium precipitant in body fluids and a cause of muscle fatigue.

Another poison prevented from release in the bowel is histamine. As a dilator of blood vessels, it can cause a histamine headache as well as bring on allergy symptoms and bloating of the colon.

For optimum nutritional value, complex carbohydrates should be eaten raw. A word of caution at this point will help avoid much intestinal distress. Although raw foods represent the highest quality carbohydrates available, an abrupt change may not be well tolerated by most people. A history of consuming primarily refined foods, increased amounts of protein, accompanied by various degrees of gastritis will in most cases decrease the body's ability to handle a high-fiber diet. A more successful transition will be made by utilizing nutritional supplements that support gastric and intestinal healing and by slowly introducing high-fiber foods that have been lightly cooked. Cooking lightly involves steaming or boiling for 3 or 4 minutes to soften the fibrous contents while still preserving most of the nutritional value. The following is recommended as an initial approach to alleviating gastritis and gastric ulcer problems.

Comfrey-pepsin capsule (recommended dosage: one capsule with each meal; in cases of acute gastritis, one capsule every half hour until pain subsides)

Gastrex capsule (recommended dosage: two capsules 15 minutes before each meal)

Zypan (recommended dosage: 1 or 2 tablets should be taken midway through each meal to help assimilate the nutrients)

These supplements are available from Standard Process Laboratories (Milwaukee, Wisconsin Tel.# [414] 933-2100). These natural supplements will provide the raw materials for stomach repair. Relief should come within 7 to 10 days. This is based on the fact that the stomach lining is completely renewed every 4 to 7 days. A period ranging from 3 months to a year or possibly longer may be required for the digestive system (including the enzyme-producing organs–pancreas, stomach, and liver, which manufactures bile for fat digestion) to adequately heal itself and to become capable of handling the more fibrous foods.

With the exception of the possible contamination by pesticides and the small percentage of deterioration due to transit time, raw foods offer the least toxicity of any substances we put in our body. A major benefit is that our organs of detoxification do not have to work as hard to keep our internal system clean. This translates into a more efficient immune system, a slower rate of degeneration and fewer illnesses. Maintaining this state of balance is achieved by eating 60 to 80 per cent alkaline-forming foods. The essential alkaline-forming elements (calcium, sodium, potassium, and magnesium) are essential for the body chemistry to maintain its acid–alkaline balance. As the cells function, a constant stream of acid waste products are released. This presents no problem as long as there is a plentiful supply of alkaline-forming elements. Crucial to the maintenance of health is the availability of calcium and sodium. Both minerals have demonstrated their ability to insure cell vitality and increase resistance against bacteria.

# FATS

Fats, also known as lipids, provide the most concentrated source of energy in the diet. When broken down, fats release 9 calories per gram (30 grams = 1 ounce). This energy release represents twice the calories furnished by either carbohydrates or proteins. The chemical structure of fats includes carbon, hydrogen, and oxygen but no nitrogen. Fats are not soluble in water. As lipids, they also function as carriers for the fat-soluble vitamins, A, D, E, and K. Fats assist the conversion of carotene to vitamin A and also enhance vitamin D absorption making calcium available to body tissues. As a whole, fats function in three main areas: (1) to insulate, protect, and support organs; (2) to participate in biochemical reactions within the body; and (3) to store additional energy.

Fats have a definite effect on the digestion of foods. When present in meals, fats will reduce stomach secretions, delaying the digestive process and the emptying time of stomach contents. This has the effect of maintaining the feeling of fullness and delaying the sensations of hunger.

Digestion of fats begins in the stomach and is completed in the small intestine where the fats are entirely absorbed. Under the influence of fat-splitting enzymes (lipases) released by the stomach, pancreas, and small intestine, the fat is broken down into triglycerides (fatty acids) and glycerols. Approximately 30 to 50 per cent of the ingested fats are converted to fatty acids while the remaining 50 to 70 per cent are eliminated as waste material. Consuming a diet high in fiber quickens the transit time of the fatty waste. However, those individuals on a high refined carbohydrate intake will have much longer transit times and constipation problems. Since the stagnating fat becomes rancid, the toxic products potentiate the chances for developing cancer of the colon as well as increasing the toxemia level of the entire body.

Aiding the process of fat digestion are the bile salts which are produced by the liver, stored in the gall bladder, and released into the small intestine. The bile salts have an emulsifying action which helps break up the fat into small droplets, and, more importantly, enables the fatty acids, cholesterol, glycerols, and other lipids to be more easily absorbed through the intestinal wall into the venous blood supply and lymphatic circulation. Once in the body, the fatty acids combine with various other chemical components to form hormones such as steroids, corticosteroids (estrogen and progesterone), fatty substances to pad the joints and form the sheathing on nerves, and phospholipids which become an integral part of the cell membranes and form a protective covering for the body's genetic codes, chromosomes.

Fat can also be manufactured from carbohydrates in the diet. Carbohydrates supply the raw materials, and conversion is dependent upon the quantity of insulin present. Eating a typical American diet which is approximately 20 per cent refined carbohydrates and 40 per cent fat will sensitize and predispose the pancreas to produce increased quantities of insulin. The blood sugar, glucose, is converted to fat in the liver and then transported to fat depots around the body. A consequence of this metabolism is an erratic blood sugar level. The lowering of the blood sugar level creates further cravings for sugar and a vicious cycle ensues.

Fats are classified as being saturated or unsaturated. The animal fats are the most frequently occurring saturated fats. They are palmitic and stearic acid. Oleic acid, also an animal fat, is a monounsaturated fat. Common examples of saturated fat are margarine, butter, cheese, shortening, lard, bacon grease and "lean meat". One of the major drawbacks of commercially processed foods with high saturated fat content is that chemical preservatives must be added to prevent rancidity.

## TOXIC WASTE REMOVAL

The lymphatic system represents the sewage system of the body. It functions primarily to remove the waste products produced by the cells then transfers these waste products to the bloodstream where they are carried to the appropriate organs of detoxification. The lymphatic vessels also dump their waste through the walls of the colon. This waste removal process functions effectively only when the colon is unobstructed by old fecal matter or excess amounts of mucoid matter. Diets high in saturated fats (such as in hamburgers, french fries, pizzas, processed lunch meats, ice cream, etc.)

serve to slow the action of the intestinal and lymphatic systems. As the waste backs up in the lymphatic vessels, a toxic environment is formed in the spaces that surround cells. Frequent consumption of the high saturated fat foods establishes a chronic toxic state. Since the spaces between the cells are congested with toxic wastes, nutrients cannot be properly supplied to the functioning cells. This whole scenario speeds up the degenerative process within the body.

## Dangerous Effects of Homogenized Milk

Studies have linked homogenized cow's milk to this country's abnormally high rate of atherosclerosis. This degenerative disease is caused by a build-up of a yellowish, fatty placque which coats the inner lining of the arterial walls, especially of the blood vessels that supply the heart muscle. The problem stems from the fact that cow's milk (but not human milk) has a high concentration of an enzyme called xanthine oxidase. This connection was brought to light by Dr. Kurt A. Oster, M.D., chief of cardiology at Park City Hospital, Bridgeport, Connecticut. Xanthine oxidase is normally present in the fat globules of milk. However, in milk that has not been homogenized, the fat globules are too large to diffuse through the intestinal wall and be absorbed by the bloodstream. The process of homogenization breaks up the fat globules into tiny droplets which can then be easily absorbed into the bloodstream. Because the American diet is so high in fats (approximately 40 per cent) arterial placque build-up starts at a very young age.

The unsaturated fats are commonly referred to as the polyunsaturated fats. They are primarily found in vegetables, nuts, seeds, corn, sesame, sunflower, safflower and fish oils. The polyunsaturates lack hydrogen atoms within their structure which enables other chemical components to become attached and form new substances. Polyunsaturates such as linoleic, linolenic, and arachidonic acid are essential fatty acids which the body cannot synthesize and must obtain from the diet to insure proper growth, reproduction, lactation, tissue repair, and hormone production. They also provide the building blocks for many biochemical essentials and help to regulate the presence of others.

Linoleic acid, for example, is the most important polyunsaturated fat in the diet because it helps to regulate the levels of cholesterol. In addition, both linoleic and linolenic acid are converted by the liver to arachidonic acid which also acts as a cholesterol-metabolizing substance. Arachidonic acid plays another vital role in that it provides the principal component in the synthesis of prostaglandins. These prostaglandins are hormone-like chemical messengers found in most cells of our body. The current physiologic concept views these substances as modulators of hormone activity, that is, the prostaglandins activate or inhibit the reactions of hormones. Although the body has an adequate supply of the polyunsaturates, a deficiency may still exist because of the presence of diabetes, liver dysfunction, old age, and impairment by the presence of other fats.

In order for these unsaturated fatty acids to be utilizable by the body, they must be in a specific biological geometric form. In basic language that means the atoms are oriented around the axis of the chemical structure in a specific manner. In the natural form it is called a *cis* configuration. However, when man begins to tamper with nature, subtle changes occur which nullify the biological activity of the original natural structure. Use of modern technology to process food (heating, hydrogenating oils to form margarine, etc.) converts the chemical structure into a *trans* configuration. From a technical standpoint both forms have the identical components but differently arranged. It is this subtle alteration that inhibits the formation of the chemical messengers and steroid hormones (sex and adrenal hormones) from the parent structure, linoleic acid.

A past professor of medicine at the University of Montreal, Dr. David Horrobin, and other reliable researchers have established the benefits of using the unsaturated fatty acid, gamma linolenic, in the treatment of many physical ailments (asthma, arthritis, premenstrual syndrome, multiple sclerosis, atopic eczema, hyperactivity, cholesterol overload, painful menses, functional cystic mastitis, obesity). Their studies have found, however, that when the *cis* form of the fatty acid is transformed into the *trans* configuration it cannot be used by the body and it also interferes with the cells' ability to absorb and incorporate the essential *cis* form. In order for the essential fatty acids to be truly effective, one should eliminate saturated fats, refined, processed, and hydrogenated oils from the diet.

The ingestion of excess amounts of all forms of fat, cholesterol, refined carbohydrates, and protein is potentially dangerous to the entire system. The many studies in the scientific literature bring to light the fact that the so called Western diet, which is comprised of over 40 per cent fat is strongly associated with all forms degenerative disease. Without exception, those societies which consume a low fat diet (less than 20 per cent), have a low prevalence of degenerative diseases. Fats, whether they be saturated or unsaturated, animal or vegetable, are implicated in the disease process. The biologic damage focuses on disturbing body metabolism which contributes to the source of degeneration. The mechanisms follow three basic avenues: (1) decreased oxygenation of tissues and organs; (2) disruption of carbohydrate metabolism; and (3) increased cholesterol and uric acid levels.

# NATURAL VITAMINS VERSUS SYNTHETIC VITAMINS

In 1897, a Dutch physician, Eijkman, working in Java, came to the realization that the oriental disease, beriberi, was caused by an incomplete diet which consisted primarily of polished rice. Eijkman's theory was that a toxin within the polished rice was responsible. It was not until 1901 that another Dutch researcher, Grijns, discovered that there was a protective and curative substance in the rice polishings. In looking back, Grijns was probably one of the first to develop the concept that disease was caused by a deficiency and that an active, protective nutrient within food could effect a cure.

Grijns' work motivated another researcher, Pekelharing to perform experiments utilizing purified foodstuffs. When these purified foodstuffs were fed to mice, initially, the mice ate well and appeared healthy, but after about 4 weeks on the diet they all died. In subsequent experiments, he was able to maintain the health of these mice by substituting raw milk or even whey for the water. Pekelharing concluded that "an unrecognized substance occurs in milk which is of paramount importance for nutrition, even in minute quantities."

In 1911, similar experiments were independently conducted by Osborne and Mendel in the United States and the same conclusions were established. Their study focused on the nutritive values of highly purified proteins isolated from various cereals. Their rats exhibited no growth or weight maintenance until protein-free milk was added to their diet. During approximately the same period, Hopkins in England and McCollum in the United States substantiated the findings of Osborne and Mendel. Casimir Funk, in 1911, isolated a crystalline substance from rice polishings that effected a cure for and prevented beriberi in pigeons. Since this substance appeared to be essential to life, he named it "vitamine."

# DEPLETED SOILS

A major misconception that has been accepted by many health professionals and a high percentage of the public is that our food supplies us with all the necessary vitamins and minerals. In a 1984 government publication, *The Red Book On Nutrition*, the United States Department of Agriculture sent out a shock wave. Independent laboratories around the United States took soil samples and analyzed their contents. Their reported findings revealed an across-the-board reduction, ranging from 25 per cent to 75 per cent, of the quantity of proteins, carbohydrates, fats, and 9 basic minerals. In addition, their study showed that the use of synthetic fertilizers caused the chromium in the soils to be bound up and unavailable to the plants. Because chromium is an essential mineral for the production of insulin, one can imagine its impact on the onset and amplification of diabetes. This government report coupled with the fact that about 70 per cent of our food is processed leaves very little doubt as to the need for taking quality nutritional food supplements.

# ADVANTAGES OF NATURAL VITAMINS OVER SYNTHETIC VITAMINS

A vitamin represents any of a number of complex organic substances (active soluble proteins, carbohydrates, essential fatty acids, and enzymes) which are metabolically and functionally interrelated and essential for normal functioning of the body. Natural vitamins, i.e., vitamins as they appear in foods, are bound to protein complexes. This enables them to be absorbed through the intestinal wall into the bloodstream. In foods, natural vitamins are always soluble to permit transport through the living system. Active, soluble bioflavonoids are always associated with natural vitamins when they appear in food. In the natural state, vitamins never appear singly but are always closely associated with other vitamins and trace minerals and act to enhance them. As present in foods, natural vitamins almost always occur in more than one form. For example, in natural yeast, vitamin B-6 is found as pyridoxine, pyridoxal and pyridoxamine.

Unfortunately man's arrogance has teamed up with "Madison Avenue" to deceive a gullible public into believing that the body does not know the difference between synthetic vitamins or synthetic fractions of vitamin complexes and naturally occurring vitamins. Dr. Casimir Funk, the discoverer of vitamins and the first to concentrate vitamin B said, "The synthetic product is less effective and more toxic." Structurally, synthetic vitamins are mirror images of natural vitamins. Although the synthetic form of the vitamin has the basic chemical pieces, its structure is different (rotated in a different direction) from its natural counterpart. Accepting the statement that there is no difference between natural and synthetic vitamins is like believing that your left hand will fit perfectly into a right-handed glove. The crystalline pure, synthetic forms of vitamins do not appear that way in nature. As examples, manmade vitamin B-6 (pyridoxine hydrochloride) does not exist in nature and pantothenic acid never appears in food as calcium pantothenate. They are less efficiently absorbed because the soluble protein bond is missing. Also lacking is the essential activating mineral which is closely linked to the vitamin's structure. When the synthetic vitamin is taken into the body, it must be rearranged and combined with the natural factors before it can actually function. Often much of the synthetic substance washes out of the body through the kidneys before any major amounts of natural, biologically active vitamins can be formed.

A food researcher, Agnes Fay Morgan Ph.D., at the University of California, reported (*Science,* vol. 93, pp. 261-262) as far back as 1941, that animals on a diet enriched with synthetic vitamins dropped dead long before other animals on an unenriched diet became ill. Dr. Morgan's warning at the time was that "... such phony enrichment might cause conditions worse than the original deficiency."

Synthetic vitamins at best, function in our body as drugs. As a prime example, high doses of ascorbic acid (synthetic vitamin C– which is made by a fermentation process in which sulfuric acid is bubbled through corn syrup) will produce an antihistamine effect. When "treating" the common cold with high doses of synthetic vitamin C, the user gets a false sense of relief because the symptoms are being masked.

In the August 1939 issue of the Journal of Nutrition, Dr. Barnett Sure reported on a study in which he fed one group of pigs twice the daily requirement of synthetic vitamin B-1. A second group of pigs was fed an equal amount of natural B-1. The results had frightening implications. The first generation offspring from those pigs fed synthetic B-1 were *all sterile.* However, all of the first generation offspring from the parents fed natural vitamin B-1 were healthy and fertile. It seems obvious from these results that synthetic vitamin B-1 is a genetic poison to pigs and potentially harmful to humans. These artificial vitamins are capable of damaging the chromosomes that are responsible for transmitting the sexual characteristics.

Genetic destruction is also appearing in humans. A 1981 report released by the University of Florida revealed some shocking observations. When average young American males were tested in 1929, their sperm counts were 100 million sperm cells per millimeter of semen. When sperm counts were taken 44 years later, in 1973, the average adult male's count had dropped to 60 million. Just seven years later, in 1980, the average sperm count dropped to an all-time low of only 20 million per millimeter.

Since the beginning of World War II (1939), "enrichment" of refined, devitalized foodstuffs such as white bread, cereals, pastas, and other flour products, became mandatory. It is interesting to note that 3 years before this, scientists discovered how to make synthetic vitamin B-1 (thiamine) from coal tar. From 1939 to present, people worldwide have received daily doses of synthetic fractions of false vitamins which are potential genetic poisons. Is the historical use of synthetic B-1 another example of "man's better living through the use of chemistry"?

Scientists, physicians, and nutritionists are becoming more alarmed by the use of synthetic vitamin and mineral supplements. Dr. David Heber, chief of clinical nutrition at the University of California at Los Angeles School of Medicine recently stated, "Americans should get their nutrients from food. Large supplement doses of single nutrients won't prevent disease, but instead will upset absorption of other nutrients." Dr. Victor Herbert of Mount Sinai School of Medicine in New York stated, "...scientists are now beginning to see toxic effects from large doses of some USP [denotes a synthetically pure substance] vitamins long considered harmless such as vitamin C (ascorbic acid) and some of the B vitamins."

In his book *A New Breed of Doctor,* Alan Nittler, M.D. describes the difference between USP vitamins and natural vitamins found in food. Dr. Nittler says "...like drugs, USP vitamins force reactions to take place in the body. Neither drug nor synthetic vitamin can be taken without paying a price, however. There is a vast difference between synthetic and natural vitamins and minerals, if the latter are truly natural. The synthetic vitamin contains one factor only, or perhaps a man-made combination of a few synthetics, which mixtures are merely a combination of the separate factors." Nittler went on to say, "USP vitamins can and sometimes do cause undesirable reactions" and "synthetics are non-natural elements which are really drugs by vitamin names."

Abram Hoffer, M.D., Ph.D. in his book *Medical Applications of Clinical Nutrition* describes the differences between vitamins and minerals in food (bonded to protein complexes) and USP (a synthetically pure, free-state chemical) vitamins and minerals. Hoffer also emphasizes the fact that isolated protein and other food fractions do not exist in food. Dr. Hoffer further commented that, "The components of food are not food. The combination of parts is not equivalent to the whole. In fact, these components do not exist free (unbonded) in nature; nature does not lay down pure protein, pure fat, or pure carbohydrate. Their molecules are interlaced in a very complex three dimensional structure (protein complex) which even now has not been fully described. Intermingled are the essential nutrients such as vitamins and minerals, again not free, but usually combined in complex molecules. Since food components are not complete foods, they should not be called food for this perpetuates the myth that these components comprise good food. They are food artifacts. It follows that when foods and artifacts are combined (USP vitamins mixed with natural base) the whole mixture becomes food artifact."

As informed consumers, we must break from the traditional pharmaceutical mentality that has led us to believe that there is no difference between synthetic and truly natural vitamins, that synthetic chemicals will function biologically the same as food and are harmless.

The structure of a natural vitamin is similar to that of an onion. Each layer represents a different part, such as enzymes, co-enzymes, anti-oxidants, and trace minerals that are essential for the whole vitamin to work properly. For example, in nature vitamin C is made up of ascorbic acid which is bound to a protein, and vitamin P (bioflavonoid) of which rutin is a biochemical relative. The activating trace mineral is copper. Supplying large doses of one or two synthetic or natural parts of a complex can be hazardous to one's health. At best, the fraction of the vitamin can only have a drug effect on the body. Ingesting megadoses of synthetic vitamin C (ascorbic acid–it's really a sugar) will lead to various serious consequences as reported in the following research:

1. Megadoses of vitamin C (ascorbic acid) can weaken red blood cells leading to their breakdown and release of hemoglobin and other contents into the surrounding fluid. (*Annual of Internal Medicine,* 82:810, 1975; *Annual of Internal Medicine,* 84:490, 1976; *Blood,* 49:471, 1977)

2. Megadoses of C (ascorbic acid) will irritate the gastro-intestinal lining. (*New England Journal of Medicine,* 285:635, 1971)

3. C (ascorbic acid) megadoses can lead to calcification in the kidney. (*Lancet,* 2:201, 1973)

4. Megadoses of vitamin C (ascorbic acid) can cause rebound scurvy which is a vitamin C deficiency. (*Canada Medical Assoc. Journal,* 93:893, 1965)

5. Megadoses of ascorbic acid (vitamin C) interfere with the normal metabolism of minerals. (*British Journal of Nutrition,* 24:607, 1970; *Journal of Laboratory Clinical Medicine,* 51:37, 1958)

6. Ascorbic acid megadoses may destroy vitamin B-12 in the blood. (*Journal of the American Medical Association,* 230:241, 1974; *American Journal of Clinical Nutrition,* 30:297, 1976)

Since synthetic ascorbic acid is hexose (a six-carbon simple sugar), consuming large doses has the great potential to adversely affect the insulin-producing cells of the pancreas. Diabetic conditions may actually worsen from large amounts of synthetic vitamin C, and those people who have a family history of diabetes may, in fact, quicken the onset of this degenerative disease.

One of the principal advocates in the use of megadoses of ascorbic acid for the treatment of acute infectious diseases and malignant degenerative states is the Nobel prize winner, Dr. Linus Pauling. In 1974, Dr. Pauling published *New Dynamics of Preventive Medicine.* Contrary to what most people believe, Dr. Pauling stated the truth about ascorbic acid. In his book he recommends taking "... pure crystalline ascorbic acid. It is made from glucose (corn syrup). What is called rose hips vitamin C is the same pure crystalline ascorbic acid with a pinch of rose hips powder added. It is almost impossible to buy ascorbic acid from a natural source. The rose hip and aserolebarus ascorbic acid is out of the same barrel from Hoffman-LaRoche, as the others, but with a pinch of rose hip powder." It cannot be overemphasized enough that **ascorbic acid is not vitamin C.** Ascorbic acid is a synthetic fraction of the biologically utilizable vitamin C complex!

Another major misconception which appears to be immortalized in cement, is that alpha- or mixed tocopherols is vitamin E. In reality what is being sold as vitamin E is only part of the anti-oxidant fraction of the whole complex. When fractions are chemically separated from their natural components they lose up to 99 per cent of their potency (*Annual Review of Biochemistry*, 1943, page 381). Compounding the problem even more is the fact that consuming chemically pure vitamin E (alpha and mixed tocopherols) in high unit doses (800 I.U. or more) reverses its effectiveness and produces the same symptoms as a deficiency which includes a loss of calcium from bones (*The Vitamins in Medicine,* p. 623 by Bicknell and Prescott, 3rd edition).

True vitamin E (concentrated from green peas, as produced by Standard Process Laboratory) is made up of five main layers plus its mineral activator, selenium. The tocopherol layer acts purely to protect the other layers of the E complex. The inner core contains a substance (xanthine) which enhances the potency of the tocopherols by as much as 50 per cent. Another internal ingredient (lipositols) is essential to convert cholesterol into vital hormones. Also present is vitamin F (unsaturated fatty acids) which helps to restore the calcium levels in the tissues and is thought by many to have anticancer properties. Another fraction of vitamin F promotes the repair of tissues and enhances the benefits of the anti-arthritic factor. The E-2 fraction works to increase the oxygen-conserving factor of the blood. By dilating the blood vessels supplying the heart (similar to nitroglycerine), E-2 allows more oxygen to reach the spastic heart muscle relieving the pain of angina. The last part of this natural vitamin package is the E-3 fraction. According to researchers, E-3 is needed to form sex hormones and helps heal stomach ulcers.

Other synthetic counterfeit vitamins often seen as "enrichments" on the package lablels of convenience foods and multiple vitamin supplements are:

1. Thiamine hydrochloride–synthetic form of B-1
2. Thiamine mononitrate–synthetic form of B-1
3. Pyrodoxine hydrochloride–synthetic form of B-6
4. Irradiated ergosterol–synthetic form of vitamin D
5. Vitamin A acetate or palmitate–synthetic vitamin A
6. Calcium pantothenate–synthetic form of pantothenic acid
7. Niacin–synthetic form of niacinamide

Whenever any food product contains these substances, the buyer had better beware!

## ROCKS AND PLASTER
## IN OUR FOODS AND VITAMINS

The consumer must also be aware of the inorganic minerals that are present in vitamin supplements and processed foods. These inorganic salts are being supplied by United States Gypsum Company and other similar industries. In the November 1985 issue of the trade journal, Food Processing U.S. Gypsum advertised calcium sulfate as "natural calcium." Their "hype" lures prospective food processors with their offer to achieve more cost-effective baking and food processing management by switching to calcium sulfate (plaster). They recommend its use for a variety of products as an enricher, whitener, stabilizer, taste improver, and coagulant, and they boast that the list goes on! Other vitamin products (such as Oscal, and Tums) utilize calcium carbonate (limestone) as the calcium source. Americans now have a choice. They can either eat plaster (calcium sulfate) or rocks (calcium carbonate) in the form of vitamins or food.

To be biologically effective, minerals must be bound to active, soluble protein complexes. Chemically pure minerals are inefficiently absorbed and utilized. They will be absorbed and enter the bloodstream only if protein complexes are available in the digestive tract. The protein complexes act as biological transporters and only in this bound form can they be distributed throughout the body.

Many supplement companies assure their consumers that their mineral products are derived from "natural sources." They proclaim vitamins derived from dolomite and oyster shell as natural. Although natural, rocks and shells do not contain minerals bound with protein complexes as they appear in food. Our bodies were not designed to handle these minerals in the uncombined forms, and in reality they are mostly rejected.

Many vitamin companies take advantage of the consumer by stating that their products are chelated, that is, organically bound. Chelated forms involve mineral gluconates which are formed by combining the mineral with gluconic acid. Gluconic acid, however, has never been found in nature to assist absorption and utilization of any nutrient. In reality, the gluconate form is a 100 per cent organic chemical and provides advertising hype but the nutrient actually hinders body usage.

For maximum transport to and absorption by body cells, biologically active minerals must be bound to an active, soluble protein complex. Unfortunately, most amino acid chelated minerals available today are produced with soy protein. The major drawback of using soy protein is that it is an inactive protein source. Other inactive proteins used to produce "organic minerals" are casein and egg albumin. These proteins are rendered insoluble during the destructive precipitation process by which they are combined with the inorganic minerals.

When searching for a high quality vitamin and mineral supplement, one should seek out a product in which the vitamins and minerals are bound to naturally active proteins in the same form as found in foods. A major source that provides all the active protein complexes bound to the vitamins and minerals is yeast. One commercially available vitamin and mineral supplement that meets all these requirements is "Foodform" (Intracell Nutrition Inc. P.O. Box 3070; Fort Lee, N.J. 07024 Tel.# 1-800-572-FOOD; in N.J. (201) 461-4660). Their products are in the same form as in natural foods. They are absorbed up to 5 times more readily and retained up to 16 times more than ordinary vitamins. Foodform vitamins are 97 per cent bonded to natural-form protein complexes so that they are metabolized like food.

**155**

Since the publication of *The Yeast Connection* in 1983 by William G. Crook, M.D., many people have become fearful of yeast in all forms. The lay person must realize that there are hundreds of species of yeast in our environment. Some of these yeasts are harmful while others are beneficial. The irrational fear that eating strains of nonliving beneficial forms can aggravate problems caused by accidental exposure to one of the harmful varieties is completely unfounded. It is just as ridiculous to warn consumers to avoid all yeast products. It is virtually impossible to avoid yeast because it is everywhere in our environment–in the air we breathe, in all our food, on our skin and on the clothes we wear.

# HEADACHE-CAUSING SUBSTANCES

Since 1940, the intake of chemical additives and preservatives has risen by 995 per cent. This does not include the air and water pollutants and the many drugs that people consume for chronic conditions. Exposure to chronic low levels of pollutants or sensitivity to synthetic compounds may in fact be the cause of many head pains and other symptoms. The following list of potential headache-causing substances is provided as a starting point for your relief:

1.**Caffeine:** Occurs naturally in tea, coffee, chocolate, and cola nuts. Caffeine is added to many nonalcoholic carbonated beverages. As an example, a 12-ounce can of Coke has 64.7 mg. of caffeine. Other examples including Pepsi, coffee, tea, Dr. Pepper, Mountain Dew and Root Beer all have a high caffeine content.

*Side effects:* Caffeine produces nervousness, insomnia, and a rapid heart beat. It also constricts blood vessels and has the potential to relieve vascular headaches. However, victims of tension headaches who continually consume caffeine in the form of ACP (aspirin, caffeine and phenacetin) tablets may develop headaches as the drug effects begin to wear off. Similarly, going "cold turkey" after drinking large quantities of coffee or tea will cause withdrawal headaches. This is often the cause of the so-called "weekend headache." Consuming large quantities of coffee during the work week with weekend abstinence will often be the cause.

2. **Sodium nitrite or nitrate:** These inorganic chemical compounds are used extensively as preservatives and color fixatives in cured meats, meat products, and in certain cured fish. Some commom examples are hot dogs, bacon, ham, and salami.

*Side effects:* Even the small amounts of nitrites and nitrates found in cured foods have the ability to dilate blood vessels and cause headaches in some people. This type of headache is usually characterized as a dull, aching pain accompanied by a flushed face and possibly a rapid pulse and lightheadedness.

3. **MSG (Monosodium glutamate):** MSG is a flavor enhancer and is manufactured from corn or wheat gluten or from sugar beet by-products. MSG is used extensively by restaurants to restore the fresh-cooked flavor when using canned and reheated foods. The following examples are given because they are usually seasoned with MSG: chicken, fish, shellfish, Chinese and Japanese foods, kosher chicken soup, matzoball and green pea soups.

*Side effects:* MSG symptoms usually develop 15 to 20 minutes after eating MSG-laced foods. Victims usually complain of numbness to both arms and the back, general weakness, and heart palpatations. Other symptoms include profuse cold sweats, tightness on both sides of the head, and a vise-like pounding, throbbing sensation in the head.The ensuing headache is a pressure or throbbing type over the temples with a sensation of a tight hatband across the forehead. People who are sensitive to MSG are usually susceptible to migraines and other vascular headaches.

4. **Alcohol and histamine:** Ingestion of both substances will severely dilate blood vessels. Red wines, in particular, may have a high histamine content and can trigger migraine and cluster headaches in susceptible individuals. The hangover headache on the morning after is the result of acetaldehyde, acetate, tannins, fusel oil and other breakdown products of alcohol that circulate in the blood and affect the arteries in the skull. The biggest offenders are brandy, bourbon whiskey, and red wines. Those individuals who have a high serum histamine level should also avoid synthetic multiple vitamins which have histidine which is converted to histamine in the body.

5. **Calcium proprionate or sodium proprionate:** These chemical substances are used as mold- and rope inhibitors in bread, rolls and other baked goods, poultry stuffing, chocolate products, processed cheeses, artificially sweetened fruit, jelly and preserves, pizza crust, and in food packaging materials.

*Side effects:* Moderate allergic reactions have been reported 4 to 18 hours after ingestion. Disturbances begin in the upper intestinal tract and end with partial or total migraine headaches. The stomach-intestinal distress symptoms are similar to gallbladder attacks and can be especially severe in individuals in whom there is a combined allergy and gallbladder ailment. When calcium proprionate is used, it destroys the enzyme that normally makes it possible for the body to assimilate any available natural calcium or calcium added through "enrichment" in bread.

6. **Tyramine:** This is a natural compound found in many foods. Tyramine will dilate blood vessels and thus is considered a potential allergenic headache-triggering substance. This natural compound is primarily found in red wines and aged cheeses. Those individuals sensative to this substance should avoid the following tyramine-high foods: Dairy products–sour cream, yogurt, ripened or aged cheeses, such as Chedder, Gruyere, Stilton, Emmentabo, Brie, Camembert, Gouda, Mozzarella, Parmesan, Provolone, Romano, Roquefort, Swiss, and Edam; fermented or pickled meats and fish–pickled herring, summer sausage, fermented sausage and other varieties, salami, bologna, pepperoni, salted fried fish, beef and chicken liver; vegetables–avocados, Italian broad beans with pods (fava beans), sauerkraut, Chinese food, onions, and lima beans; alcoholic beverages–beer, ále, red wines (Chianti is the worst!), Riesling, sauterne, champagne and sherry; miscellaneous–yeast and yeast extracts, chocolate, vanilla, soy sauce, and anything pickled or marinated.

7. **Foods high in salt content:** Ingestion of large amounts of salty foods will result in salt overload on the vascular system. Salt (sodium chloride) has the ability to expand the blood volume and cause the cells to retain fluids. Besides increasing blood pressure, the arteries must dilate to accommodate the additional fluid. Chronic headache sufferers, especially individuals prone to migraine and vascular head-

aches should avoid foods high in salt. Examples of high salt content foods are pork, lard, salted potato chips, crackers, salted nuts, and bacon. Also be sure to check food labels for salt content.

8. **Drugs:** Ninety per cent of the drugs listed in the *Physician's Desk Reference* (PDR) have headaches listed as one of the side effects. One must consider any medication presently being taken as a possible triggering substance. Caution must be exercised in this area since headaches must be listed as a side effect even if a very small percentage of test patients experience the symptoms.

Victims of chronic headaches or those with frequent tension headaches may be creating their own head pain by abusing the analgesic drugs being consumed. Withdrawal headaches very often can be attributed to the rebound effect of the caffeine present in the compounds. Caffeine, like nicotine, constricts the blood vessels. Going "cold turkey", either from stopping smoking or discontinuing the headache relief pills will result in dilation of blood vessels and triggering of a headache. Heavy consumption of coffee, tea and/or cigarettes on a daily basis will maintain the blood vessels in a constricted state. Failure to meet your daily quota of these substances may trigger a rebound headache.

9. **Birth control pills:** The "Pill" changes the female hormone balance. As a result, migraine-prone women usually suffer more severe headaches, while migraine-free women become more susceptible to headache pain than the nonpill user. In addition, birth control pills will reduce the vitamin B-12, folic acid, and vitamin C levels in the body.

10. **Carbon dioxide build up:** Some people habitually sleep with their heads under the sheets. Sleeping in this manner causes a build up of carbon dioxide which can cause a nasty headache upon awakening.

11. **Fluoride:** The 1983 Physicians' Desk Reference cautions: "...in hypersensitive individuals, fluorides occasionally cause skin eruptions such as atopic dermatitis, eczema, or uticaria. Gastric distress, headache, and weakness have also been reported. These hypersensitive reactions usually disappear promptly after discontinuation of the fluoride."

# Part V

# Manipulation And Healing

# STRUCTURAL CORRECTION

"THE DOCTOR OF THE FUTURE WILL GIVE NO MEDICINE BUT WILL INTEREST HIS PATIENTS IN THE CARE OF THE HUMAN FRAME, IN DIET, AND IN THE CAUSE AND PREVENTION OF DISEASE."

This profound statement was made by one of the most creative and ingenious minds of the world, Thomas A. Edison.

Structural correction as a means of healing had its beginning in September of 1895. It was Daniel David Palmer, a self-educated man from Davenport, Iowa, who discovered a principle which was used as far back as the Egyptian, Incan and other advanced civilizations. D.D. Palmer ingeniously applied a method previously unknown to correcting ills that had plagued man. This historic event occurred when Dr. Palmer restored the hearing of a Negro porter who had been deaf for 17 years. This miraculous result was accomplished by Dr. Palmer's locating and correcting an anatomical malrelationship of the fourth thoracic vertebra in his spine.

"In recent years, allopathic (traditional) medicine has been 'discovering' chiropractic and its literature, and professional journals have been replete with references to vertebral disrelations, or subluxations, and credit given to the interference of the segmental nerves by such distortion as the cause of many and diverse symptoms..." (from *The Neurodynamics of the Vertebral Subluxation* by A.E. Homewood, D.C., 1977). As a dentist, this author has also "discovered" chiropractic as it interrelates one's body to one's teeth and bite and vice versa. Although physiologic dentists throughout the world represent a minority, they have achieved greater degrees of treatment success working with chiropractic physicans. These elite dental-chiropractic teams have repeatedly demonstrated the influences of tooth position and bite on the cranium, spine, pelvis and their relationship to many physiologic disturbances such as high blood pressure, blood sugar irregularities, menstrual problems, allergies, chronic fatigue, hearing loss, delayed healing, balance problems, constipation, swollen glands (lymph nodes), eye pains, migraine headaches, etc.

As a branch of the healing arts and sciences, chiropractic focuses on the concept of the triad of health: structural, mental, and chemical. It is believed that all health problems, whether functional or pathological, are involved with one part or all of the triad. The chiropractic physician who employs this concept increases his ability to uncover the patient's underlying problem.

The well-trained chiropractic physician knows that treatment of the patient's problem may involve nutritional support, when indicated, to assist his structural manipulations and enhance the correction. He also understands the tremendous overlaying influences mental problems can have on structural imbalances as well as being a major contributing factor in causing muscle spasms, indigestion, generalized toxicity, under- or over-active glands, etc. The coordinated efforts of the professional team will focus on uncovering the underlying causes of the patient's problem. Once the main areas that are not working properly are discovered, an intelligent approach to healing can be made.

Dr. George Goodheart appropriately summed up healing when he stated, "Man possesses a potential for recovery through the innate intelligence of the human structure. This recovery potential with which he is endowed merely waits for the chiropractic hand, heart and mind to bring it to potential being and allow the recovery to take place which is man's natural heritage."

The well-educated chiropractic physician will have training in many different techniques. As with any profession, there is no one approach that will provide a cure-all. A good chiropractor will spend the necessary time to question the patient about the main complaints and then perform a thorough examination. Such an evaluation may include the cranium, spine, pelvis, and extremities. The purpose of such an evaluation is to determine the integrity of the structures and their function. To assist in diagnosing the problem, the patient may be requested to have spinal or pelvic x-rays, blood studies, urinalysis, nutritional analysis, and when necessary, a medical evaluation from a competent physician.

# Part VI

# International Physician
# Referral Directory

# International Physician Referral Directory

The following referral directory includes physicians from the various healing professions. The purpose of the directory is to offer the reader a starting point in the search for health. The professional services provided by these practitioners may be a source of relief from chronic headaches and related problems that previously have gone undiagnosed by traditional medicine practitioners.

Additional chiropractic physicians may be located by contacting the following source:

Current *International Directory of Chiropractors Trained in the Sacro Occipital Technic:*

Dr. Major B. DeJarnette
722½ Central Avenue
Nebraska City, NE 86410
(402) 873-6769

## ALABAMA

**EVERS HEALTH CENTER**
**H. RAY EVERS, M.D.**
600 Mineral Wells Road
P.O. Box 587
Cottonwood, Al 36320
(205) 691-2161
MEDICAL: All Chronic Degenerative Diseases, Nutritional Counseling

**GREEN SPRINGS CHIROPRACTIC CENTER**
**JOHN A. FARMER DC**
2156 Green Springs Hwy.
Birmingham, Al 35205,
(205) 251-1251
CHIROPRACTIC: Sacro Occipital Technique, TMJ, Cranial Manipulation, Nutritional Counseling, Physio-therapy, Musculo-Skeletal Reeducation

## ALASKA

**G.S. KHALSA, D.C.**
308 Fifth Avenue
Fairbanks, Ak 99701
(907) 456-2244
CHIROPRACTIC: Applied Kinesiology, Sacro Occipital Technique, Nutrition, Holistic Approach

**WILLIAM R. RISCH, D.C.**
440 W. Tudor Road
Anchorage, Ak 99503
(907) 563-3839
CHIROPRACTIC: Sacro Occipital Technique, Nutritional Counseling, Cranial Manipulation

**RICHARD NEWMAN, D.C.**
**DEBORAH KLOBY, D.C.**
703 W. Northern Lights
Anchorage, Ak 99503
(907) 274-8605
CHIROPRACTIC: Atlas Orthogonnal, Toftness, Activator Extremity Cranial, Chiromanis, Applied Kinesiology

**JOHN R. KEIFER, D.C.**
899 N. Wilmot
# A-4
Tucson, Az 85711
(602) 327-3777
CHIROPRACTIC: Applied Kinesiology,
Diversified Activator, Cox, Nutrition,
Acupuncture

**ELIZABETH AHLES, D.C.**
21 W. Baseline Road
Tempe, Az 85283
(602) 839-9040
CHIROPRACTIC: Palmer, Kinesiology,
Physical Therapy, Nutrition

**R.C. MASSNER, D.C.**
2063 Thumb Butte Road
Prescott, Az 86301
(602) 445-4390
CHIROPRACTIC: Spinal, Cranial, Extremities, Therapy Sports Injuries, Nutritional Counseling

**THOMAS R. DEMERS, D.C.**
1907 W. Union Hills Drive
Phoenix, Az 85023
(602) 993-1916
CHIROPRACTIC: Peirce Stillwagon, Sacro Occipital Technique, Diversified, Logan Basic, Gonstead, Nutrition

**A.R.E. CLINIC**
**DRS. WILLIAM and GLADYS McGAREY**
4018 N. 40th Street
Phoenix, Az 85018
(602) 955-0551
MEDICAL: Traditional/Holistic, Biofeedback, Massage, Colonics, Stress Management, Dreamwork, Hypnotherapy, Color Therapy, Brain Injury Program involving Patterning

**SHELDON C. DEAL, D.C.**
1001 N. Swan Rd.
Tucson, AZ 85711
(602) 323-7133
CHIROPRACTIC: Applied Kinesiology,
Cranial Manipulation, TMJ, Nutritional
Counseling

**JOHN W. BRIMHALL, D.C.**
901 8th Ave.
Holbrook, AZ 86025
(602) 524-6855
CHIROPRACTIC: Applied Kinesiology,
Cranial Manipulation, Nutritional Counseling

**ROBERT PLANT, D.D.S.**
25 Arch Street
Redwood City, Ca 94062
(415) 368-7291
DENTAL: TMJ

**DAVID G. DENTON, D.C.**
12381 Wilshire Blvd.
Los Angeles, Ca 90025
(213) 826-6664
CHIROPRACTIC: Sacro Occipital Technique, Applied Kinesiology, Craniopathy, TMJ, Extremity Work, Nutritional Counseling

**HAROLD E. RAVINS, D.D.S.**
12381 Wilshire Blvd. Ste.103
Los Angeles, Ca 90025
(213) 207-4617
DENTAL: TMJ, Dental Orthopedics,
Orthodontics, Nutritional Counseling

**CURTIS C. BUDDINGH, D.C.**
22114 Ventura Blvd
Woodland Hills, Ca 91364
(818) 704-4255
CHIROPRACTIC: Sacro Occipital Technique, Applied Kinesiology, Cranial Manipulation, TMJ, Extremity Work, Dyslexia, Learning Disabilities, Nutritional Counseling

**MARC G. PICK, D.C.**
206 S. Robertson Blvd.
Beverly Hills, Ca 90211
(213) 655-1420
CHIROPRACTIC: Sacro Occipital Technique, Craniopathy, TMJ, Applied Kinesiology, Extremity Work, Nutritional Counseling

**STANLEY Y. INOUYE, D.D.S.**
5931 Stanley Ave.
Carmmichael, Ca 95608
(916) 392-5670
DENTAL: TMJ, Dental Orthopedics,
Orthodontics

**DWIGHT JENNINGS, D.D.S.**
P.O. Box 877
17 S. Buena Vista
Ione, Ca 95640
DENTAL: TMJ, Dental Orthopedics,
Orthodontics, Nutritional Counseling

**DEAN BOWMAN, D.C.**
19963 Ventura Blvd.
Woodland Hills, Ca 91364
(818) 340-8950
CHIROPRACTIC: Palmar, Logan Basic,
Pain Control, Meric, Applied Kinesiology

**ROBERT DERRYBERRY, D.C.**
6050 Third Street
Ventura, Ca 93003
(805) 656-3737
CHIROPRACTIC: Sacro Occipital Technique, Gonstead, Applied Kinesiology

**STEWERT BLAIKIE, D.C.**
6050 Third Street
Ventura, Ca 93003
(805) 656-3737
CHIROPRACTIC: Gonstead, Sacro Occipital Technique, Diversified, Specific

**GEORGE PETOW, D.C.**
672 Thousand Oaks Blvd
Thousand Oaks, Ca 91360
(805) 495-8786
CHIROPRACTIC: Applied Kinesiology, Diversified, Nutrition

**ANDREA WILLIAMS, D.C.**
1055 Sunnyvale-Saratoga Road
Sunnyvale, Ca 94087
(408) 730-2202
CHIRPRACTIC: Applied Kinesiology, Sacro Occipital Technique, Diversified

**INES and BRUCE FREEDMAN, D.C.**
617 Cherry Chase Ctr
Sunnyvale, Ca 94087
(408) 739-2161
CHIROPRACTIC: Full Spine, Diversified, Gonstead, Sacro Occipital Technique, Aplied Kinesiology

**MARTIN FALLICK, D.C.**
1055 Sunnyvale-Saratoga Road
Sunnyvale, Ca 94087
(408) 737-0730
CHRIROPRACTIC: Diversified, Applied Kinesiology

**REBECCA WEST, D.C.**
1743 Grand Cannal
Stockton, Ca 95207
(209) 477-5159
CHIROPRACTIC: Diversified, Applied Kinesiology, Cranial, Nutrition

**JAMES ADAMS, D.C.**
101 Andrieux Street
Sonoma, Ca 95476
(707) 996-4535
CHIROPRACTIC: Sacro Occipital Technique, Applied Kinesiology, Cranial

**SUSAN UDRY, D.C.**
1203-A Washington Ave.
Santa Monica, Ca 90403
(213) 393-6806
CHIROPRACTIC: Sacro Occipital Technique, Applied Kinesiology, Activator, Nutrition, Diversified, Physical Therapy

**ROBERT MORRIS, D.C.**
1243 7TH Street
Santa Monica, Ca 90401
(213) 451-5851
CHIROPRACTIC: Applied Kinesiology, Full Spine, Nutritional Counseling, Physical Therapy

**TARAS LUMIERE, D.C.**
2105 Wilshire Blvd.
Santa Montica, Ca 90403
(213) 829-0453
CHIROPRACTIC: Applied Kinesiology, Activator, Acupuncture, Nutrition

**HARVEY MARKOVITZ, D.C.**
1830 Commercial Way
Santa Cruz, Ca 95065
(408) 476-7344
CHIROPRACTIC: Applied Kinesiology, Diversified, Activator, Nutrition

**SANDRA LINWOOD, D.C.**
2116 Soquel Ave.
Santa Cruz, CA 95062
(408) 425-5777
CHIROPRACTIC: Sacro Occipital Technique, Applied Kinesiology, Cranial, Nutrition, Homeopathy

**JERALD ADAMS, D.C.**
1290 Scott Blvd.
Santa Clara, Ca 95050
(408) 247-4640
CHIROPRACTIC: Applied Kinesiology, Full Spine, Gonstead

**DANIEL WAGNER, D.C.**
40 E. Alamar
Santa Barbara, Ca 93105
(805) 682-2407
CHIROPRACTIC: Sacro Occipital Technique, Diversified, Activator, Physical Therapy, Acuscope

**RAYMOND CASTELLINO, D.C.**
106 W. Mission
Santa Barbara, Ca 93101
(905) 569-1216
CHIROPRACTIC: Sacro Occipital Technique, Cranial Manipulation, TMJ, Activator, Spinal Stress, Nutritional Counseling

**JACOB BASTOMSKI, D.C.**
1625 State Street
Santa Barbara, Ca 93101
(805) 569-5000
CHIROPRACTIC: Applied Kinesiology, COX, Diversified, Thompson, Physical Therapy

**168**

**MARC JOHNSTON, D.C.**
1150 Grove Street
P.O. Box 1918
San Luis Obispo, Ca 93406
(805) 541-2727
CHIROPRACTIC: Sacro Occipital Technique, Gonstead, Straight

**WRIGHTMONT PROFESSIONAL CENTER**
MARILYN STAHL, D.C.
990 W. Fremont Ave.
Suite T
San Jose, CA 94083
(408) 947-8186
CHIROPRACTIC: Sacro Occipital Technique, Activator, Diversified

**MITCHELL PEARCE, D.C.**
100 O'Connor Dr. #3
San Jose, Ca 95133
(408) 294-2424
CHIROPRACTIC: Sacro Occipital Technique, Cranial, Diversified, Nutrition, COX, Physical Therapy

**JEAN REVERE, D.C.**
220 Bush Street #450
San Francisco, Ca 94104
(415) 434-1530
CHIROPRACTIC: Sacro Occipital Technique, Applied Kinesiology, Motion Palpation

**THOMAS McDONALD, D.C.**
607 Market Street 3rd Fl
San Francisco, Ca 94105
(415) 546-6906
CHIROPRACTIC: Sacro Occipital Technique, Nimmo, Physical Therapy, Nutrition

**JOSEPH MANISCALCO, D.C.**
3210 Fillmore Street
San Francisco, Ca 94123
(415) 346-0363
CHIROPRACTIC: Gonstead, Physical Therapy, Nutrition, TMJ, Cranial, Acuscope, Diversified

**JAMES SILVA, D.C.**
750 Kains Ave.
San Bruno, Ca 94066
(415) 952-3080
CHIROPRACTIC: Sacro Occipital Technique, Applied Kinesiology, Gonstead, Activator, Diversified, Nutritional Counseling

**CARL FELT, D.C.**
9426 Magnolia Ave.
Riverside, Ca 92503
(714) 688-0104
CHIROPRACTOR: Sacro Occipital Technique, Gonstead, Activator

**NELSON FELDMAN, D.C.**
1816 Tribute Rd.
Sacramento, Ca 95815
(916) 925-8934
CHIROPRACTIC: Applied Kinesiology, Non Force, Cox, Nutritional Counseling

**PATRICIA GAYMAN, D.C.**
1065 W. Cypress Ave.
Redding, Ca 96001
(916) 241-1872
CHIROPRACTIC: Sacro Occipital Technique, Activator, Holistic Health Services

**JO ANN DOROTHY, D.C.**
780 E. Green Street
Pasadena, Ca 91101
(818) 795-7617
CHIROPRACTIC: Sacro Occipital Technique, Applied Kinesiology, Activator, Diversified, Physical Therapy

**JOHN CULLEN, D.C.**
21 S. Roosevelt Ave.
Pasadena, Ca 91107
(818) 796-4866
CHIROPRACTIC: Sacro Occipital Technique, Applied Kinesiology, Cranial, TMJ, Palmer, Logan, Diversified

**CHRISTOPHER HARRISON, D.C.**
299 California #200
Palo Alto, Ca 94306
(415) 326-1003
CHIROPRACTIC: Applied Kinesiology, Sacro Occipital Technique, Spinal Stress, Gonstead, Activator, Nutritional Counseling

**ALEXANDER EDISS, D.C.**
490 S. Farrell #C-102
Palm Springs, Ca 92262
(619) 323-7600
CHIROPRACTIC: Applied Kinesiology, Nutrition, Diversified, Physical Therapy

**JOHNATHAN LEMIER, D.C.**
1259 W. Gonzales Rd.
Oxnard, Ca 93030
(805) 485-1802
CHIROPRACTIC: Sacro Occipital Technique, Applied Kinesiology, Cranial Manipulation, Diversified, Nutrition

**CATHERINE KLEIBER, D.C.**
300 S. Fifth Street
Oxnard, Ca 93030
(805) 483-6636
CHIROPRACTIC: Sacro Occipital Technique, Applied Kinesiology, Gonstead, Acuscope

**STEVEN CSER, D.C.**
172 N. Tustin Ave.
Orange, Ca 92667
(714) 532-6881
CHIROPRACTIC: Sacro Occipital Technique, Diversified, Gonstead, Activator, Nutritional Counseling

**VICTOR TOMASSETTI, D.C.**
2741 Vista Way #111
Oceanside, Ca 90254
(619) 757-0222
CHIROPRACTIC: Sacro Occipital Technique, Applied Kinesiology, Diversified

**TODD ADAMS, D.C.**
4121 Westerly Pl #116
Newport Beach, Ca 92660
(714) 752-5753
CHIROPRACTIC: Sacro Occipital Technique, Diversified, Activator, Gonstead, Nutritional Counseling, Physical Therapy

**JAMES NICHOLS, D.C.**
1042 Country Club Dr.
Moraga, Ca 94556
(415) 376-7080
CHIROPRACTIC: Applied Kinesiology, Gonstead, Activator, Nutritional Counseling

**MICHAEL WEIR, D.C.**
530 Ramona
Monterey, Ca 93940
(408) 372-5602
CHIROPRACTIC: Sacro Occipital Technique, Applied Kinesiology, Cox, Activator, Diversified, Nutritional Counseling

**JEFFREY FOUNTAIN, D.C.**
1077 Cass Street
Monterey, Ca 93940
(408) 373-5636
CHIROPRACTIC: Applied Kinesiology, Gonstead, Activator

**JAY OSBORNE, D.C**
1917 Coffee Rd.
Medesto, Ca 95355
(209) 524-5214
CHIROPRACTIC: Applied Kinesiology, Full Spine, Diversified

**CHARLES KUNTZ, D.C.**
9919 Sepulveda Blvd.
Mission Hills, Ca 91345
(818) 894-4077
CHIROPRACTIC: Applied Kinesiology, Homeopathy, Diversified, Activator, Total Body Modification

**PHINA McBRIDE, D.C.**
4519 Admiralty Way
Marina Del Ray, Ca 90292
(213) 827-5567
CHIROPRACTIC: Sacro Occipital Technique, Cranial Manipulation, Diversified

**RALPH HOYT, D.C.**
1150 W. Center St. #104
Manteca, CA 95336
(209) 239-3593
CHIROPRACTIC: Applied Kinesiology, Sacro Occipital Technique, Cranial Manipulation, Nutritional Counseling, Diversified

**PETER PAULAY, Ph.D., D.C.**
103 Gilbert Ave.
Nenlo Park, CA 94025
(415) 323-6374
CHIROPRACTIC: Directional Non-Force Technique, Bio-magnetic Resonance Analysis, Nutritional Analysis, Yeast Infections (Candida), Sports Injuries, Allergies

**CARL ROTHSCHILD, D.C.**
**NEAL SNYDER, D.C.**
2365 Westwood Blvd.
Los Angeles, CA 90064
(213) 475-9111
CHIROPRACTIC: Diversified/F.S., Cox, Applied Kinesiology, Physical Therapy, Sports, Nutrition

**AKASHA KHALSA, D.C.**
**HARI KHALSA, D.C.**
**SATCHARN KHALSA, D.C.**
**WAHEGURU KHALSA, D.C.**
1536 S. Robertson Blvd.
Los Angeles, CA 90035
(213) 274-8291
CHIROPRACTIC: Sacro Occipital Technique, Nutrition, Cranial, Yoga Therapy, Applied Kinesiology

**PAUL M. HOLT, D.C.**
2904 Rowena Ave.
Los Angeles, CA 90039
(213) 660-2370
CHIROPRACTIC: Diversified Full Spine, Applied Kinesiology, Nutrition

**DONALD FLUEGEL, D.C.**
6317 Wilshire Blvd.
#401
Los Angeles, CA 90048
(213) 852-4984
CHIROPRACTIC: Diversified, Nutrition, Applied Kinesiology, Activator, Physical Therapy, Cox, F/SP

**MICHAEL BILLAUER, D.C.**
3223 Washington Blvd.
Los Angeles, CA 90292
(213) 306-1983
CHIROPRACTIC: Sports Med., Applied
Kinesiology, Diversified/F.SP., Cox, Physical Therapy

**APRIL MODESTI, D.C.**
1178 Los Alto Ave.
Los Altos, CA 94022
(415) 949-1089
CHIROPRACTIC: Applied Kinesiology,
Sacro Occipital Technique, Activator

**LINDA NELSON, D.C.**
1 Larkspur Plaza Dr.
Larkspur, CA 94939
(415) 927-1040
CHIROPRACTIC: Full Spine, Applied
Kinesiology, Sports Med., Exercise Equipment, Physical Therapy, Aquatic Therapy,
Extremities, Vidio Analysis

**ROBIN ALEXANDER, D.C.**
3462 Mt. Diablo Blvd.
Lafayette, CA 94549
(415) 283-8140
CHIROPRACTIC: Sacro Occipital Technique, Applied Kinesiology, Diversified,
Nutrition

**D.J. VAN DYCK, D.C.**
3011 Honolulu
La Crescenta, CA 95719
(818) 249-4226
CHIROPRACTIC: Palmer, Logan, Applied
Kinesiology

**NEDDA ROVELLI, D.C.**
810 Healdsburg Ave.
Healdsburg, CA 95448
(707) 433-2955
CHIROPRACTIC: MP Analysis, Diversification, Gonstead, Sacro Occipital Technique, Deep Tissue

**DEBORAH KARISH, D.C.**
810 Healdsburg Ave.
Healdsburg, CA 95448
(707) 433-2955
CHIROPRACTIC: MP Analysis, Diversified, Gonstead, Sacro Occipital Technique,
Deep Tissue

**MICHAEL OLFF, D.C.**
1303 A St.
Hayward, CA 94541
(414) 889-8171
CHIROPRACTIC: Diversified, Applied
Kinesiology, Activator, Sacro Occipital
Technique

**RICHARD SMITH, D.C.**
317 N. Verdugo Rd.
Glendale, CA 91206
(818) 246-1704
CHIROPRACTIC: Diversified, Sacro Occipital Technique, Gonstead, Best, Spinal
Touch, Applied Kinesiology, Orthopedist,
Laser Acupuncture, Roentgenologist

**RITA SCHROEDER, D.C.**
**THOMAS SCHROEDER, D.C.**
2535 N. Fresno
Fresno, CA 93703
(209) 226-2535
CHIROPRACTIC: Diversified, Kinesiology, Sacro Occipital Technique

**KENNETH RITTER, D.C.**
1046 E. Shields Ave.
Fresno, CA 93704
(209) 226-1048
CHIROPRACTIC: Applied Kinesiology,
Thompson, Best, Diversified

**R. STEVEN HOOPES, D.C.**
2053 N. Fresno St.
Fresno, CA 93703
(209) 222-7796
CHIROPRACTIC: Palmer, Gonstead,
Applied Kinesiology, Nutrition

**PATRICIA HANSEN, D.C.**
445 N. McPhersonn St.
Ft. Bragg, CA 95437
(707) 964-7566
CHIROPRACTIC: Diversified, Applied
Kinesiology, Physical Therapy, Nutrition

**DOUGLAS HETRICK, D.C.**
201 E. Grand St.
#1-C
Escondido, CA 92025
(619) 741-0774
CHIROPRACTIC: Applied Kinesiology,
Cranial, Chiromanis

**SUE GOLDBERG, D.C.**
803 E. Grand Ave.
Escondido, CA 92025
(714) 746-7401
CHIROPRACTIC: Diversified Full Spine,
Electro Acupuncture, Spinal Touch, Applied
Kinesiology, Reflex Techniques, Physical
Therapy

**DAVID WELLS, D.C.**
5363 Balboa Blvd.
3234
Encino, CA 91316
(818) 788-4220
CHIROPRACTIC: Applied Kinesiology,
Activator, Nutrition, Physical Therapy

**ROBERT S. EBERLE, D.C.**
22762 Aspan
#201
El Toro, CA 92630
(714) 770-5052
CHIROPRACTIC: Applied Kinesiology,
Activator, Cranial, Diversified

**JOSEPH and CAROL BALL, D.C.**
10164 San Pablo Ave.
El Cerrito, CA 94530
(415) 525-8611
CHIROPRACTIC: Sacro Occipital Technique

**JOHN E. BAUM, D.C.**
450 Fletcher Parkway
#201
El Cajon, CA 92020
(619) 588-2002
CHIROPRACTIC: Diversified, Gonstead,
Extremities, Cranial, TMJ, Applied Kinesiology, Acutherapy, Nutrition

**RICHARD PALASKI, D.C.**
3550 Willow Pass Rd.
Concord, CA 94519
(415) 676-8200
CHIROPRACTIC: Gonstead, Cox, Activator, Sacro Occipital Technique

**DORIS MEGGET, D.C.**
1123 Briarcroft Rd.
Claremont, CA 91711
(714) 624-4719
CHIROPRACTIC: Sacro Occipital Technique, Activator, Applied Kinesiology,
Nutrition

**DUANE W. COX, D.C.**
6104 Greenback Lane
Citrus Heights, CA 95626
(916) 723-3977
CHIROPRACTIC: Sacro Occipital Technique, Gonstead, Child Treatment

**PARADISE CHIROPRACTIC**
LINDA BERRY, D.C.
1700-A Solano Ave.
Berkeley, CA 94707
(415) 526-6657
CHIROPRACTIC: Light Force Applied
Kinesiology, Nutrition, Craniopathy, Sacro
Occipital Technique, Live Cell Blood
Analysis

**PATRICIA WILSON, D.C.**
849 First St.
Benicia, CA 94510
(707) 746-1200
CHIROPRACTIC: Sacro Occipital Technique, Activator, Muscle Work, Renaissance

**SMITH-WOLFF CHIROPRACTIC GROUP**
WILSON E. SMITH, D.C.
1437 Seventh St.
Suite 301
Santa Monica, CA 90401
(213) 458-8020
CHIROPRACTIC: Applied Kinesiology,
Cranial Manipulation, Nutritional Counseling

**THIE CHIROPRACTIC CLINIC**
JOHN F. THIE, D.C.
1192 N. Lake Ave.
Pasadena, CA 91104
(818) 798-7805
CHIROPRACTIC: Applied Kinesiology,
TMJ, Touch for Health, Sports Injuries

**RUEGER-POWERS CHIROPRACTIC INC.**
DRS. DALE H. POWERS
JANET L. RUEGER
1534 Solano Ave.
Albany, CA 94707
(415) 526-4394
CHIROPRACTIC: Sacro Occipital Technique, Motion Palpation, TMJ, Cranial
Manipulation, Nutritional Counseling,
Macrobiotic Information, Sports Injuries
Rehabilitation

**DIRECTOR-TOLWCAN CHIROPRACTIC**
VINCENT P. SAVARESE, D.C.
North Hollywood, CA 91601
(818) 769-1811
CHIROPRACTIC: Applied Kinesiology,
Chiropractic Orthopedics, Nutritional
Counseling

**CHERYL JOY BRATMAN, D.C.**
2432 Lincoln Blvd.
Suite A
Santa Monica, CA 90405
(213) 392-9795
CHIROPRACTIC: Sacro Occipital Technique, Applied Kinesiology, Cranial Manipulation, Nutritional Healing, TMJ,
Acupressure

**CHARLES L. BLUM, D.C.**
2432 Lincoln Blvd.
Suite A
Santa Monica, CA 90405
(213) 392-9795
CHIROPRACTIC: Sacro Occipital Technique, Applied Kinesiology, TMJ, Cranial
Manipulation, Nutritional Healing

**VIRGINIA I. HANDLY, D.C.**
14428 Union Ave.
San Jose, CA 95124
(408) 377-6931
CHIROPRACTIC: Sacro Occipital Technique, Cranial Manipulation, Nutritional
Healing, Applied Kinesiology

**ANDERSON CHIROPRACTIC CENTER**
MARY B. ANDERSON, D.C.
503 N. HWY 101
Solana Beach, CA 92075
(619) 755-8055
CHIROPRACTIC: Recurrent Headache Therapy, Chronic Low Back and Leg Pain, Nutritional Healing, Applied Kinesiology, Electro Acupuncture

**BRUCE BADDOE, D.C.**
881 Alma Real #316
Pacific Palisades, CA 90272
(213) 454-0648
CHIROPRACTIC: Nutritional Coounseling, Applied Kinesiology, Cranial Manipulation, Non-Force Adjusting, Holistic Approach

**ROBERT M. BLAICH, D.C.**
12301 Wilshire Blvd.
Suite 416
W. Los Angeles, CA 90025
(213) 820-7320
CHIROPRACTIC: Applied Kinesiology

**ROBERT J. PESHEK, D.D.S.**
7759 California Ave.
Riverdale, CA 92504
(714) 688-2733
DENTAL: TMJ Dysfunction, Cranio-Facial Pain, Nutritional Counseling

## COLORADO

**LINDA HALTEMAN, D.C.**
**DAVID CRISTE**
434 Oak St.
Steamboat Springs, CO 80477
(303) 879-1845
CHIROPRACTIC: Sacro Occipital Technique, Activator, Nutrition, Stress Management

**ROGER DRUCKMAN, D.D.S.**
1555 S. Havana St.
Auroro, CO 80012
(303) 751-7773
DENTAL: Orthodontics, TMJ, Orthopedics

**LINDA HALTEMAN, D.C.**
**DAVID CRISTE**
434 Oak St.
Steamboat Springs, CO 80477
(303) 879-1845
CHIROPRACTIC: Sacro Occipital Technique, Activator, Nutrition, Stress Management

**LOUISVILLE CHIROPRACTIC HEALTH CENTER**
LINDA KLEIN, D.C.
1032 S. Boulder Rd. #205
Louisville, CO 80027
(303) 666-7887
CHIROPRACTIC: Toftness, Activator, Sacro Occipital Technique

**ROBERT MASTELLER, D.C.**
917 S. Main
Longmont, CO 80501
(303) 651-1886
CHIROPRACTIC: Toftness, Activator, Gonstead, Applied Kinesiology, Nutrition, Sacro Occipital Technique

**DONALD JOHNSTON, D.C.**
2255 Mountain View Ave.
Longmont, CO 80501
(303) 772-5042
CHIROPRACTIC: F.SP., Thompson, Applied Kinesiology, Activator, Logan Basic

**ALFRED EUHUS, D.C.**
6650 S. Vine St.
Littleton, CO 80121
(303) 794-5192
CHIROPRACTIC: Activator, Cox, Applied Kinesiology, Diversified

**MARK WOLFF, D.C.**
345 S. Union Blvd.
Lakewood, CO 80228
(303) 986-5122
CHIROPRACTIC: Applied Kinesiology, Sacro Occipital Technique, Nutrition, Orthopedics

**GOLDEN CHIROPRACTIC AND HOLISTIC HEALTH CENTER**
FAYE STEPHENSON, D.C.
JOHN T. UNGER
2600 East St.
Golden, CO 80401
(303) 278-3678
CHIROPRACTIC: Applied & Clinical Kinesiology, Sports Injuries, Cox, Acupuncture, Nutrition Assessment & Therapy & Digestion Problems, PMS, Candida, Allergies, Neurologic & Orthopedic Problems

**GLENN BARNETT, D.C.**
6941 Hwy. 73
Evergreen, CO 80517
(303) 670-1815
CHIROPRACTIC: Applied Kinesiology, Sacro Occipital Technique, Activator, Nutrition

**DAVID RAWLINGS, D.C.**
7090 E. Hamden
Denver, CO 80224
(303) 759-2468
CHIROPRACTIC: Applied Kinesiology, Sacro Occipital Technique, Diversified, Acupuncture, Nutrition

**JOHN FISHER, D.C.**
16135 S. Golden Rd.
Denver, CO 80401
(303) 278-8188
CHIROPRACTIC: Activator, Applied Kinesiology, Diversified, Nutrition

**DAVID ACKERMAN, D.C.**
601 Broadway
#317
Denver, CO 80203
(303) 592-1571
CHIROPRACTIC: Diversified, Applied Kinesiology, Nutrition, Acupuncture

**JAMES WAYNE, D.C.**
201 S. Wilcox
Castle Rock, CO 80104
(303) 688-9133
CHIROPRACTIC: Sacro Occipital Technique, Diversified, Nutrition, Physiotherapy

**DAVID VORZIMER, D.C.**
**DAVID MAMOLEN, D.C.**
724 Pearl St.
Boulder, CO 80302
(303) 449-3103
CHIROPRACTIC: Low Force, Sacro Occipital Technique, Activator, Diversified

**THOMAS PATTERSON, D.C.**
17200-L E. Lliff Ave.
Aurora, CO 80013
(303) 750-3280
CHIROPRACTIC: Applied Kinesiology, Diversified, Lab, Nutrition, Psysiotherapy

**TERESA SALVADORE, D.C.**
135 W. Main
Aspen, CO 81611
(303) 920-1247
CHIROPRACTIC: Applied Kinesiology, Diversified, Acupuncture, Nutrition

**STEPHEN J. KAUFMAN, D.C.**
6300 E. Yale
Suite 105
Denver, CO 80224
(303) 759-4594
CHIROPRACTIC: Applied Kinesiology, Nutritional Counseling, Sacro Occipital Technique, Acupuncture

**FAYE M. STEPHENSON, D.C.**
2600 E. St.
Golden, CO 80401
(303) 278-3678
CHIROPRACTIC: Applied Kinesiology, Nutritional Therapy, Macrobiotics, Acupuncture, Massage Therapy, Bach Flower Remedies

**GARY N. KLEPPER**
1440 28th
Boulder, CO 80302
(303) 449-7388
CHIROPRACTIC: Applied Kinesiology, Clinical Kinesiology, Clinical Nutrition, Acupuncture, Botonical Medicine, Cranial Manipulation, TMJ

# CONNECTICUT

**NEW HAVEN CRANIOFACIAL PAIN CENTER**
PAUL ERLANDSON
STANTON FATER
JOAN C. FAULKNER
ROBERT SORRENTINO
1423 Chapel St.
New Haven, CT 06511
(203) 787-6581
DENTAL-PHYSICAL THERAPY: TMJ, Sacro Occipital Technique, Cold Laser Therapy, Physical Therapy, Oral Surgery, Biofeedback

**JOAN C. FAULKNER, R.P.T**
116 S. Main St.
Wallingford, CT 06492
(203) 265-0018
PHYSICAL THERAPY: TMJ, Cold Laser Therapy, Physical Therapy, Sacro Occipital Technique, Myofacial Release Techniques

**PAUL MILLER, D.C.**
27 Chestnut Hill Rd.
Norwalk, CT 06857
(203) 846-3424
CHIROPRACTIC: Diversified, Applied Kinesiology, Nutrition, Physical Therapy

**STEVEN LEONTI, D.C.**
1353 Boston Post Rd.
Madison, CT 06443
(203) 245-1666
CHIROPRACTIC: Diversified, Applied Kinesiology, Activator, Cox Nutrition, Physical Therapy

**KAREN SHIELDS, D.C.**
56 Lafayette Pl.
Greenwich, CT 06830
(203) 629-2727
CHIROPRACTIC: Applied Kinesiology, Sacro Occipital Technique, Activator, Nutrition, Physical Therapy, DNFT, Stressology, Sports, Scoliosis

**VINCENT BUONANNO, D.C.**
219 Milbank Ave.
Greenwich, CT 06830
(203) 661-6699
CHIROPRACTIC: Diversified, Sacro Occipital Technique, Applied Kinesiology, Physical Therapy, Nutrition, Cox

**174**

**BEDDING HOLISTIC CHIROPRACTIC**
BRICE and MARILYN BICKELY, D.C.
727 Redding Rd.
W. Redding, CT 06896
(203) 938-9000
CHIROPRACTIC: Applied Kinesiology,
Electro Acupuncture According to Voll,
Colonic Therapy, Nutritional and Gland-
ular Testing, Body and Foot Massage,
Barium Bowel X-Rays

## DELAWARE

**ALBERT W. FORWOOD, D.C.**
6 Sharpley Rd. & Concord Pike
Wilmington, DE 19803
(302) 652-0411
CHIROPRACTIC: Full Spine, Gonstead,
Activator, Sacro Occipital Technique,
Nutrition

**BRUCE H. CARRICK, D.C.**
**KEN DE GROOT**
3600 Silverside Rd.
Wilmington, DE 19810
(302) 478-1443
CHIROPRACTIC: Sacro Occipital Tech-
nique, Craniopathy, Diversified, F.SP.,
Extremity/Athletic Injury

**THOMAS ASHE, D.C.**
721 Philadelphia Pike
Wilmington, DE 19809
(302) 764-5668
CHIROPRACTIC: Activator, Full Spine,
Diversified, Applied Kinesiology

**ALLEN CHIROPRACTIC**
RODGER C. ALLEN, D.C.
322 N. Governors Ave.
Dover, DE 19901
(302) 734-9824
CHIROPRACTIC: Sacro Occipital Technique, Allergies, Chiropractic Manipulative Reflex Technique, TMJ, Cranial
Manipulation

**DANIEL ROSE-REDWOOD, D.C.**
918 16th St. N.W.
#100
Washington, Washington, D.C. 20006
(202) 466-3803
CHIROPRACTIC: Motion Palpation,
Thompson, Sacro Occipital Technique,
Palmer

## DISTRICT OF COLUMBIA

**LARRY BROWN, D.C.**
1330 New Hampshire Ave.
#114
Washington, Washington, D.C. 20036
(202) 887-6787
CHIROPRACTIC: Sacro Occipital Technique, Applied Kinesiology, Gonstead,
Diversified, Full Spine

## FLORIDA

**CARL DAFFIN, D.D.S.**
1394 Timberlane Rd.
Tallahassee, FL 32312
(904) 893-5462
DENTAL: TMJ

**ABDEL-FATTAH, D.D.S.**
315 Golfview Dr.
Suite 216
Boca Raton, FL 33432
(305) 391-5331
DENTAL: TMJ, Holistic Approach

**SPORTS PHYSICAL THERAPY, INC.**
DANIEL F. GOLDSTEIN, P.T.
1896 Palm Beach Lakes Blvd. No. A
West Palm Beach, FL 33409
(305) 478-2322
PHYSICAL THERAPY: Physical Therapy, Myofacial Release Techniques, TMJ

**DAVID H. HOCK, D.D.S.**
4040 Newberry Rd.
Suite 1200
Gainesville, FL 32607
(904) 376-3400
DENTAL: TMJ

**DALE A. BARNES, D.C.**
316 Church St.
Kissimmee, FL 32741
(305) 847-8254
CHIROPRACTIC: Sacro Occipital Technique, Craniopathy, TMJ, Diversified

**JAMES VANDENBERGHE, D.D.S.**
3200 S. Madison St.
New Port Richey, FL 33552
(813) 849-0705
DENTAL: TMJ, Orthodontics, Dental
Orthopedics, Myofacial Release Techniques

**RICHARD A. WINANS, D.C.**
6836 Ridge Rd.
Port Richey, FL 33568
(813) 847-5900
CHIROPRACTIC: Applied Kinesiology,
Cranial Manipulation, TMJ

**THE UPLEDGER INSTITUTE**
DR. JOHN E. UPLEDGER
11211 Prosperity Farms Rd.
Palm Beach Gardens, FL 33410
(305) 622-4334
OSTEOPATHIC: Cranial Osteopathy,
Biofeedback, Psychotherapy, Acupuncture,
Psychosomatic Medicine, Osteopathic Ma-
nipulation

**ROBERT SMITH, D.C.**
1550 Sixth St. S.E.
Winter Haven, FL 33880
(813) 293-8836
CHIROPRACTIC: Diversified, Gonstead,
Sacro Occipital Technique, Receptor Tonus,
Applied Kinesiology, Physical Therapy,
Acupuncture

**ALICE MELLOW, D.C.**
1225 W. 45th St. #307
West Palm Beach, FL 33407
(305) 842-3500
CHIROPRACTIC: Diversified, Physiotherapy, Nutrition, Applied Kinesiology

**LOUIS KLIONSKY, D.C.**
1401 S. Military Trail
West Palm Beach, FL 33415
(305) 439-4900
CHIROPRACTIC: Full Spine, Applied
Kinesiology, Sacro Occipital Technique

**DANIEL PLA, D.C.**
1907 W. Sligh Ave.
Tampa, FL 33604
(813) 935-7125
CHIROPRACTIC: Diversified, NIMMO,
Physical Therapy, Applied Kinesiology,
Nutrition, Gonstead

**MICHAEL HERRING, D.C.**
700 W. Waters Ave.
Tampa, FL 33604
(813) 932-5391
CHIROPRACTIC: Palmer Diversified,
Sacro Occipital Technique, Gonstead

**RICHARD CLANCY, D.C.**
2162 Gulf Gate Rd.
Sarasota, FL 33581
(813) 923-3424
CHIROPRACTIC: COX, Activator, Sacro
Occipital Technique, Diversified, Physical
Therapy, Nutrition, Sports and Personal
Injuries

**JAMES KINSEY, D.C.**
3137 49th St. N.
St. Petersburg, FL 33710
(813) 525-8881
CHIROPRACTIC: Gonstead, COX, Applied Kinesiology

**BENJAMIN KAUFMAN, D.C.**
7710 N.W. 56th Way
Pompano, FL 33067
(305) 428-7100
CHIROPRACTIC: Applied Kinesiology,
Diversified, Nutrition, Activator, Physical
Therapy

**FRANK PUREELI, D.C.**
6250 Park Blvd.
Pinellas Park, FL 33565
(813) 541-2520
CHIROPRACTIC: PST, Thompson, Gonstead, Diversified, Physical Therapy,
Applied Kinesiology, Activator

**ALLAN K. FRASURE, D.C.**
P.O. Box 347
Live Oak, FL 32060
(904) 362-3400
CHIROPRACTIC: Applied Kinesiology,
Cranial Manipulation, Gonstead, Palmer,
Diversified, Nutritional Counseling, Nutri-
tional Therapy

**DWAIN D, NORWOOD, D.C.**
440 N. Cove Blvd.
Panama City, FL 32401
(904) 785-8511
CHIROPRACTIC: Gonstead, Motion Palpation, Applied Kinesiology, Specific

**WALTER BAUMAN, D.C.**
3613 Highway 231
Panama City, FL 32404
(904) 785-8311
CHIROPRACTIC: Activator, Applied
Kinesiology, Nutrition

**GARRY DULGAR, D.C.**
Maitland Ave. and Ballard St.
Orlando, FL 32701
(305) 293-9663
CHIROPRACTIC: Diversified, NIMMO,
Logan Basic, Thompson, COX, Applied
Kinesiology, Nutrition

**JOHN TOWNS, D.C.**
1820 Park Ave.
Orange Park, FL 32073
(904) 264-2988
CHIROPRACTIC: Sacro Occipital Technique

**DENIS GULLIVER, D.C.**
720 S. Volusia Ave.
Orange City, FL 32763
(904) 775-3223
CHIROPRACTIC: Full Spine Diversified,
Activator, Sacro Occipital Technique,
Physical Therapy

**JEFFREY PITTS, D.C.**
801 N.E. 25th Ave.
Ocala, FL 32670
(904) 732-0200
CHIROPRACTIC: Grostic, Gonstead, Thompson, Sacro Occipital Technique, Diversification

**PHILLIP LEON, D.C.**
18545 N.E. 18th Ave.
N. Miami Beach, FL 33179
(305) 940-6161
CHIROPRACTIC: Diversified, Reflexology, Sacro Occipital Technique, Certified, Sports Injury, Acupuncture

**MARLIN COKER, D.C.**
97 Ninth St. N.
Naples, FL 33940
(813) 262-2290
CHIROPRACTIC: Diversified, COX, Activator, Sacro Occipital Technique, Thompson, Physical Therapy

**LEE BARBACH, D.C.**
7166 Pembroke, Rd.
Miramar, FL 33023
(305) 981-2225
CHIROPRACTIC: COX, Activator, Thompson, Sacro Occipital Technique

**MICHAEL BAUM, D.C.**
**WILBUR WISHNER**
1175 71st St.
Miami Beach, FL 33141
(305) 864-1419
CHIROPRACTIC: Diversified, Physiotherapy, Nutrition, Applied Kinesiology

**KENDALL LAKES CHIROPRACTIC CENTER**
MARK HOFFMAN, D.C.
13500 N. Kendall Dr. #175
Miami, FL 33186
(305) 385-0044
CHIROPRACTIC: Diversified Full Spine, Applied Kinesiology, COX, Gonstead, Nutrition, Modalities

**JEFFREY GREENBERG, D.C.**
8905 S.W. 87th Ave.
Miami, FL 33176
(305) 279-2222
CHIROPRACTIC: Palmer, Gonstead, Physical Therapy, Nutrition, Applied Kinesiology

**ERIC COHEN, D.C.**
9211 Bird Rd.
Miami, FL 33165
(305) 552-7655
CHIROPRACTIC: Gonstead, Applied Kinesiology, COX, Nutrition, Acupuncture, Physical Therapy

**JAY GUTIERREZ, D.C.**
500 N. Harbor City Blvd.
Melbourne, FL 32935
(305) 254-2367
CHIROPRACTIC: Cranial, Sacro Occipital Technique, Gonstead, Applied Kinesiology, Nutrition, Acupuncture, Physical Therapy, Palmer

**LYLE FLEMING, D.C.**
31 E. Nelson Ave.
Melbourne, FL 32935
(305) 254-2367
CHIROPRACTIC: F/SP, Sacro Occipital Technique, Activator, Physical Therapy, Acupuncture

**M. I. GARFINKLE, D.C.**
6000 Kimberly Blvd.
Margate, FL 33068
(305) 975-0200
CHIROPRACTIC: Diversified Full Spine, Activator, Applied Kinesiology, Physical Therapy, Nutrition

**NORMAN LISABETH, D.C.**
5548 W. Oakland Park Blvd.
Lauderhill, FL 33313
(305) 733-9455
CHIROPRACTIC: Applied Kinesiology, Diversified, Nutrition, Physiotherapy, Ambutrak

**JERRY TANKERSLEY, D.C.**
516 W. Dixie
P.O. Box 1288
Lake Worth, FL 33460
(305) 582-7462
CHIROPRACTIC: Sacro Occipital Technique, Applied Kinesiology, Gonstead, Nutrition, TMJ, Equilibration

**LAURENCE SEIGLER, D.C.**
194 Country Club Rd.
Lake Mary, FL 32746
(904) 323-6626
CHIROPRACTIC: Palmer Full Spine, Applied Kinesiology, Thompson, NIMMO

**PAMELA GREENE, D.C.**
4414 Florida National Dr.
Lakeland, FL 33803
(813) 644-8451
CHIROPRACTIC: Applied Kinesiology, Activator, Diversified

**POMPANO BEACH CHIROPRACTIC CLINIC**
REVIS B. CHESHIRE, D.C.
4 N.E. 4th Ave.
Pompano Beach, FL 33060
(305) 943-1044
CHIROPRACTIC: Sacro Occipital Technique, Cranial Manipulation, Vitamin Therapy, Nutritional Counseling, Extremity Adjusting, TMJ

MICHAEL CHANCE, D.C.
1225 N.W. 10th Ave.
Gainesville, FL 32601
(904) 375-6972
CHIROPRACTIC: Special Upper Cervical, Thompson, Applied Kinesiology, Sacro Occipital Technique, Nutrition

ROBERT ROGOFF, D.C.
6991 W. Broward Blvd.
Ft. Lauderdale, FL 33317
(305) 583-1901
CHIROPRACTIC: Diversified, Applied Kinesiology, Physical Therapy

PETER FISHMAN, D.C.
1730 E. Commercial Blvd.
Ft. Lauderdale, FL 33334
(305) 771-1940
CHIROPRACTIC: Diversified F.SP., Extremities, Sacro Occipital Technique, COX, NIMMO, Applied Kinesiology, Gonstead, Nutrition, Activator

MARC FELDMAN, D.C.
8039 W. Oakland Park Blvd.
Ft. Lauderdale, FL 33321
(305) 748-4445
CHIROPRACTIC: Activator, Sacro Occipital Technique, COX Chiromanis, Diversified

DAVID BERNSTEIN, D.C.
997 E. Oakland Park Blvd.
Ft. Lauderdale, FL 33334
(305) 565-4440
CHIROPRACTIC: Applied Kinesiology, Kinesiology, Acupuncture, COX, Thompson, Diversified, Physiotherapy

JOHN GAFFNEY, D.C.
339 E. New York Ave.
Deland, FL 32724
(904) 734-4490
CHIROPRACTIC: Gonstead, Motion Palpation, Nutrition, Acupuncture, Applied Kinesiology, Nautilus Rehabilitation

W.R. MUNSTER, D.C.
229 Second St.
Daytona, FL 32017
(904) 258-1034
CHIROPRACTIC: Gonstead, COX, Sacro Occipital Technique

DENNIS GOLDEN, D.C.
7832 W. Sample Rd.
Coral Springs, FL 33065
(305) 752-4000
CHIROPRACTIC: Sacro Occipital Technique, Full Spine, Gonstead

JAMES WOOD, D.C.
1121 53rd. Ave. West
Bradenton, FL 33507
(813) 753-3441
CHIROPRACTIC: Full Spine, Diversified, Gonstead, Sacro Occipital Technique

ROBERT CANELLI, D.C.
1518 53rd Ave.
P.O. Box 1551
Bradenton/Oneco, FL 33558
(813) 758-2666
CHIROPRACTIC: Activator, Sacro Occipital Technique, Grostic, Palmer, Acupuncture

RONALD PLUESE, D.C.
4799 N. Federal Highway
Boca Raton, FL 33431
(305) 395-8100
CHIROPRACTIC: Diversified Full Spine, Physical Therapy, Activator, Applied Kinesiology, Nutrition

MICHAEL MARSHALL, D.C.
4331 N. Federal Highway
Boca Raton, FL 33431
(305) 391-2221
CHIROPRACTIC: Applied Kinesiology, Sacro Occipital Technique, Harmonics, Acupuncture

STEPHEN BLUM, D.C.
2200 W. Glades Rd./Glades Plaza
Boca Raton, FL 33431
(305) 368-3338
CHIROPRACTIC: Full Spine, Diversified, All Therapies, Applied Kinesiology, Nutrition

KEVIN CONNELL, D.C.
366 S. Main St.
Belle Glade, FL 33430
(305) 996-1976
CHIROPRACTIC: Applied Kinesiology, TBM, Versendal, Allergies, Nutrition

MAX M. WEAVER, D.D.S.
One Doctors Lane
Lake Wales, FL 33853
(813) 676-8536
DENTAL: TMJ, Chronic Headaches and Facial Pain

DE CAMP CHIROPRACTIC
DRS. NELSON and CAMERON DE CAMP
206 Easton Drive
Lakeland, FL 33803
(813) 686-3011
CHIROPRACTIC: Sacro Occipital Technique, Nutritional Healing, Cranial Manipulation, TMJ (Coordinate Therapy with Dentists), Holistic Approach

## LEO B. STOUDER, D.C.
1926 Hollywood Blvd.
Suite 105
Hollywood, FL 33020
(305) 922-9355
CHIROPRACTIC: Applied Kinesiology, Activator Adjustments (Non-Force Technique), Nutritional Counseling, Acupuncture

## McCORD CHIROPRACTIC CENTER
KERRY M. McCORD, D.C.
6110 9th St. N.
St. Petersburg, FL 33703
(813) 522-5511
CHIROPRACTIC: Applied Kinesiology, Nutritional Counseling, Acupuncture, Physical Therapy, Cardiovascular Fitness Evaluation, X-Ray

## OWEN CHIROPRACTIC CLINIC PA
DR. L. THORNTON OWEN, Jr.
4331 Lakeworth Ave.
Lakeworth, FL 33461
(305) 965-5600
CHIROPRACTIC: Sacro Occipital Technique, Endocardiology, Vascular Evaluation, Herbs, Natural Healing (Glandular and Chelation Therapy), Structural and Muscular Corrections, Applied Kinesiology

## CHARLES ROBERT VICKERS, D.C.
4325 Highland Park Boulevard
Lakeland, FL 33803
(813) 644-5541
CHIROPRACTIC: Sports Injury Analysis, Physical Therapy, Cranial Manipulation, Sacro Occipital Technique, Nutritional Counseling - Vitamin Therapy, Applied Kinesiology, Radiology

## KIRK M. CRIST, D.C.
320 5th Ave. S.
Naples, FL 33940
(813) 262-0606
CHIROPRACTIC: Nutritional Blood Analysis, Live-Blood Analysis, Applied Kinesiology, Acupuncture, Massage Therapy, Preventive Therapeutics

## LEE N. SHELDON, D.M.D.
2223 Sarno Rd.
Melbourne, FL 32935
(305) 259-9980
DENTAL: Nutritional Counseling, TMJ and Facial Pain, Holistic Approach

## RALPH GARCIA JR., D.D.S.
2110 W. Buffalo
Tampa, FL 33607
(813) 872-4402
DENTAL: TMJ, Cranio-Facial Pain, General Dentistry

# GEORGIA

## JUSTIN L. JONES, D.D.S.
3485 Northside Parkway, N.W.
Suite 105 - Standard Federal Bldg.
Atlanta, GA 30327
(404) 237-1512
DENTAL: TMJ, Dental Orthopedics

## LANCE CHIROPRACTIC CENTER
SANDRA M. LANCE, D.C.
3960 Peachtree Rd. Suite 400
Atlanta, GA 30319
(404) 233-4433
CHIROPRACTIC: Sacro Occipital Technique, TMJ

## STEVEN BARNETT, D.C.
5385 Five Forks Trickum Rd.
Stone Mountain, GA 30087
(404) 923-7966
CHIROPRACTIC: Diversified, COX, Applied Kinesiology, Sacro Occipital Technique, Activator

## STEVEN SAUL, D.C.
225 Redfern Village
St. Simons Island, GA 31522
(912) 638-7850
CHIROPRACTIC: Sacro Occipital Technique, Applied Kinesiology, Full Spine, Nutrition, Physical Therapy

## CHARLES CROCKER, D.C.
611 S. Lee St.
Kingsland, GA 31548
(912) 729-5644
CHIROPRACTIC: Sacro Occipital Technique, Gonstead

## STEVEN WEINIGER, D.C.
1355 Frontage Rd.
Conyers, GA 30208
(404) 922-8150
CHIROPRACTIC: Applied Kinesiology, Sacro Occipital Technique, Diversified, Physical Therapy

## RONALD and ALAN WEINSTEIN, D.C.
1536 Monroe Dr. #4
Atlanta, GA 30324
(404) 892-8191
CHIROPRACTIC: Activator, Applied Kinesiology

## ATLANTA FAMILY CHIROPRACTIC CENTER
WILLIAM SAYER, D.C.
5075 Roswell Rd. #124
Atlanta, GA 30342
(404) 256-1161
CHIROPRACTIC: Ful Spine Diversified, Physical Therapy, COX, Sacro Occipital Technique, Applied Kinesiology, NIMMO

**VIRGINIA MAYO, D.C.**
375 Pharr Rd. N.E. #102
Atlanta, GA 30305
(404) 237-1707
CHIROPRACTIC: Applied Kinesiology,
Diversified, Holistic

**LINDA LEE, D.C.**
375 Pharr Rd. N.E. #102
Atlanta, GA 30305
(404) 237-1707
CHIROPRACTIC: Applied Kinesiology,
Diversified, Full Spine, Holistic Clinic

**NED GLADSTONE, D.C.**
**LARRY HABERSKI, D.C.**
3201 Tucker-Norcross Rd.
Atlanta, GA 30084
(404) 496-1375
CHIROPRACTIC: F.SP. Diversified,
Applied Kinesiology, HIO, Thompson,
COX, Pierce, Nutrition

**RUSSELL FORGOSTON, D.C.**
7268 Roswell Rd.
Atlanta, GA 30328
(404) 394-7733
CHIROPRACTIC: Full Spine, Thompson, Diversified, NIMMO, Logan Basic,
Applied Kinesiology

**WALTER BEAUMONT III, D.C.**
4166 Newton Drive
Covington, GA 30209
(404) 787-6113
CHIROPRACTIC: Applied Kinesiology,
Nutrition, Sports Injuries

**G. KEVIN ROBINSON, D.C.**
2758 Chamblee-Tucker Rd.
Atlanta, GA 30341
(404) 457-1508
CHIROPRACTIC: Chiropractic Atlas
Orthogonal Technique, Chiropractic Orthopedics

**LARRY L. TILLEY, D.D.S.**
300 Piedmont St.
Calhoun, GA 30701
(404) 629-0131
DENTAL: TMJ, General Dentistry, Mercury Free Fillings, Physical Therapy

**WILLIAM B. WILLIAMS, D.M.D.**
1147 S. Hairston Rd.
Stone Mountain, GA 30083
(404) 292-8622
DENTAL: TMJ, General Dentistry, Mercury Free Fillings, Nutritional Counseling

**HAWAII**

**OGAWA CHIROPRACTIC, INC.**
976-1 Kuhio Highway
Kapaa Kauai, HI 96746
(808) 822-7113
CHIROPRACTIC: Sacro Occipital Technique, Palmer Package, Best, Logan

**LAWRENCE CONNORS, D.C.**
45-1144 Kam Highway
Kaneohe, HI 96744
(808) 235-6677
CHIROPRACTIC: Applied Kinesiology,
Full Spine, Activator, COX, Nutrition

**MICHAEL J. SMITH, D.C.**
1314 S. King St.
#661
Honolulu, HI 96814
(808) 536-4668
CHIROPRACTIC: Full Spine, Diversified, Applied Kinesiology, Physical Therapy, COX Flexion Technique, Sports
Injuries

**GEORGE CLEMENS, D.C.**
1631 Kapiolani Blvd.
#202
Honolulu, HI 96814
(808) 955-1122
CHIROPRACTIC: Full Spine, Diversified,
Applied Kinesiology, Sacro Occipital Technique, COX, Physical Therapy

**IDAHO**

**MICHAEL MORIARTY, D.C.**
3113 Overland Rd.
Boise, ID 83705
(208) 343-3022
CHIROPRACTIC: Applied Kinesiology,
Diversified, Activator, Nutrition

**ILLINOIS**

**SAMUEL PERVA, D.C.**
210 Skokie Valley Rd.
Highland Park, IL 60035
(312) 831-5252
CHIROPRACTIC: Sacro Occipital Technique, Craniopath, TMJ

**HOMER K. MANOLIS, D.D.S.**
48 E. 31st St.
Lagrange, IL 60525
(312) 352-6811
DENTAL: TMJ, Functional Orthodontics

**ALLYNE ROSENTHAL, D.C.**
30 S. Michigan Ave.
Suite 500
Chicago, IL 60603
(312) 782-3762
CHIROPRACTIC: Sacro Occipital Technique

**IEVA WRIGHT, D.D.S.**
30 S. Michigan Ave.
Suite 500
Chicago, IL 60603
(312) 236-3226
DENTAL: TMJ

**RAYMOND HATLAND, D.D.S.**
5701 N. Ashland
Chicago, IL 60660
(312) 334-4166
DENTAL: TMJ, Cranial Osteopathic
Manipulation, Nutritional Counseling

**NOEL LAPP, D.D.S.**
6827 W. 171st St.
Tinley Park, IL 60477
(312) 532-1184
DENTAL: TMJ

**ROBERT SCHMISSEUR, D.D.S.**
111 S. State St.
Champaign, IL 61820
(217) 359-1911
DENTAL: TMJ

**GRIFFITH PRITCHARD, D.D.S.**
2807 N. Knoxville
Peoria, IL 61604
(309) 682-1213
DENTAL: TMJ

**SIGNAL HILL MEDICAL BLDG.**
MICHAEL DYER, D.D.S.
10200 W. Main St.
Belleville, IL 62223
(618) 397-2464
DENTAL: TMJ

**WELLSPRING CHIROPRACTIC CENTER**
JENNA EISENBERG, D.C.
CRAIG HILGENDORF, D.C.
1425 N. Main St.
Wheaton, IL 60187
(312) 668-9626
CHIROPRACTIC: Applied Kinesiology,
Nutrition, Diversified

**CALVIN TOKUMOTO, D.C.**
416 E. Ogden St. #D
Westmont, IL 60559
(312) 789-2030
CHIROPRACTIC: Applied Kinesiology,
Physical Therapy, Diversified

**COLLEEN KENNEDY, D.C.**
416 Ogden Ave. #D
Westmont, IL 60559
(312) 789-2030
CHIROPRACTIC: Applied Kinesiology,
Polarity, Acupuncture, Nutrition, Physical
Therapy

**DOUGLAS TRAVEN, D.C.**
915 W. Wise Rd.
Schaumburg, IL 60193
(312) 893-0390
CHIROPRACTIC: Lab, Physical Therapy, Acupuncture, Kinesiology, Nutrition

**EDWIN T. JACH, D.D.S.**
5 Plaza
Park Forest, IL 60466
(312) 748-4222
DENTAL: General Dentistry, Mercury
Free Fillings, Nutritional Counseling,
Acupuncture

**CHARLES J. HEER, D.C.**
2000 W. Pioneer Pkwy.
Peoria, IL 61615
(309) 692-2242
CHIROPRACTIC: Acupuncture, Nutrition, Blood Analysis, Allergies, Physical
Therapy, Applied Kinesiology

**WILLIAM D. HANKINS, D.C.**
MEDICAL ARTS BLDG.
1101 Main St.
Peoria, IL 61606
(309) 676-2242
CHIROPRACTIC: Nutrition, Applied
Kinesiology, F.SP., Activator, Physical
Therapy, Blood/Hair Analysis

**DONALD and NANCY SELVIDGE, D.C.**
608 Broadway
P.O. Box 943
Mattoon, IL 61938
(217) 235-4664
CHIROPRACTIC: Activator, Applied
Kinesiology, Nutrition, Physical Therapy

**GEORGE CLINIC OF CHIROPRACTIC**
SHIRL E. GEORGE, D.C.
1802 W. Irving Park Rd.
Hanover Park, IL 60103
(312) 837-8900
CHIROPRACTIC: Lab, Physical Therapy, X-Ray, Full Spine, Acupuncture,
Kinesiology, Spinal Angular Traction

**MARK ENSWELLER, D.C.**
2861 Central St.
Evanston, IL 60201
(312) 864-0411
CHIROPRACTIC: NIMMO, Diversified,
COX, Sacro Occipital Technique, Physical
Therapy

**LESTER HOLZE, D.C.**
2000 Larkin Ave. #200
Elgin, IL 60120
(312) 888-4770
CHIROPRACTIC: Applied Kinesiology,
Activator, Lab, Nutrition, Homeopathy,
Biomagnetic, Acupuncture, Holistic

**DANIEL LUBAN, D.C.**
425 W. Front St.
El Paso, IL 61738
(309) 527-2840
CHIROPRACTIC: Grostic, HIO, Sacro
Occipital Technique

**NANCY CLARK, D.C.**
1401 E. Oakton St.
Des Plaines, IL 60018
(312) 635-6664
CHIROPRACTIC: Toftness, Thompson,
Acutherapy, Applied Kinesiology, Physical
Therapy, Nutrition, Vascular Analysis,
Lab, X-Ray

**ROBERT PULS, D.C.**
46 E. Superior
Chicago, IL 60611
(312) 944-7857
CHIROPRACTIC: Diversified Full Spine,
Gonstead, Applied Kinesiology, Nutrition,
Physical Therapy

**SANDRA SCHWARTZ, D.C.**
206 Burwash
Champaign, IL 61874
(217) 351-2021
CHIROPRACTIC: Basic, Thompson, Activator, Acupuncture, Applied Kinesiology,
Diversified

**WILLIAM D. HANKINS, D.C.**
1704 E. Emmpire
Bloomington, IL 61701
(309) 662-1666
CHIROPRACTIC: Nutrition, Applied
Kinesiology, F.SP. Activator, Physical
Therapy, Blood/Hair Analysis

**DRS. POHUNEK & WINTERNHEIMER,
D.C.**
7008 W. Cermak Rd.
Berwyn, IL 60402
(312) 795-7040
CHIROPRACTIC: Gonstead, Kinesiology

**FONDER HEALTH CENTER**
AELRED CHARLES FONDER, D.D.S.,
F.A.P.D., F.A.F.P.
303 W. 2nd St.
Rock Falls, IL 61071
(815) 625-0346/0384
DENTAL: Orthodontics, Dental Ortho-
pedics, Applied Kinesiology, Sacro Occipital
Technique, Splint Therapy, TMJ

**WELLSPRING CHIROPRACTIC
CENTER**
JENNA EISENBERG, D.C.
CRAIG HILGENDORG, D.C.
1425 N. Main St.
Wheaton, IL 60187
(312) 668-9626
CHIROPRACTIC: Applied Kinesiology,
Nutritional Counseling, Clinical Kinesi-
ology, Natural Childbirth Classes, Merid-
ian Therapy, Sports Injury

## INDIANA

**PHILIP JONES, D.D.S.**
1035 N. 9th St.
Clinton, IN 47842
(317) 832-3531
DENTAL: TMJ

**DAVID G. LEHMAN, D.D.S.**
1444 Olive St.
Elkhart, IN 46514
(219) 264-9934
DENTAL: TMJ

**RANDALL A. SCHMIDT, D.D.S.**
7891 Broadway
Merrillville, IN 46410
(219) 769-6691
DENTAL: TMJ

**ROBERT MCMAHON, D.D.S**
8691 Connecticut St.
Merrillville, IN 46410
(219) 769-2720
DENTAL: TMJ

**LEWIS MYERS, D.C.**
2403 Campbell
Valparaiso, IN 46383
(219) 464-4444
CHIROPRACTIC: Applied Kinesiology,
Toftness, Activator, Thompson, COX

**DONALD DANKLEFSEN, D.C.**
P.O. Box 159
Kendallville, IN 46755
(219) 347-1637
CHIROPRACTIC: Applied Kinesiology,
COX Chiromanis, Gonstead, NIMMO,
Nutrition, Physical Therapy

**TRI STATE CHIROPRACTIC CLINIC**
J.L. SOUDER, D.C.
R.R.2, Box 774
Angola, IN 46703
(219) 665-3106
CHIROPRACTIC: Nutrition, Pierce, Ki-
nesiology, Spinal Touch, Physical Therapy,
COX, Truscott, Reams

IOWA

**EUGENE SHAY, D.C.**
**JEFFREY SHAY**
1300 Cedar St.
Muscatine, IA 52761
(319) 263-7235
CHIROPRACTIC: Sacro Occipital Technique, Basic, Diversified, Physical Therapy, Nutrition

**GENE ZDRAZIL, D.C.**
1401 Franklin St.
Iowa City, IA 52240
(319) 337-9366
CHIROPRACTIC: Sacro Occipital Technique, NIMMO, Applied Kinesiology, Activator

**BURLINGTON CHIROPRACTIC CENTER**
FORREST HEISE, D.C.
2930 Division St.
Burlington, IA 52601
(312) 754-6081
CHIROPRACTIC: Applied Kinesiology, Diversified, Thompson, Nutrition, Physical Therapy

**MERLE D. BEAN, D.D.S.**
UNIVERSITY CHILDREN'S DENTISTRY
2900 University, Suite f-3
West Des Moines, IA 50265
(515) 225-3585
DENTAL: TMJ, Cranio-Facial Pain, Dental Orthopedics, Orthodontics

KANSAS

**ALLEN THOMAS, D.C.**
9703 W. 63rd Terrace
SHAWNEE MISSION, KS 66203
(913) 831-4545
CHIROPRACTIC: Applied Kinesiology, Certified Orthopedist, Full Spine

**PARMELE CHIROPRACTIC OFFICE**
JAMES L. PARMELE, D.C., D.I.C.S.
305 N. Minnesota
Columbia, KS 66725
(316) 429-2661
CHIROPRACTIC: Sacro Occipital Technique, Ultra Sound Therapy

KENTUCKY

**FLOYD FISH, D.C.**
4011 Taylor Blvd.
Louisville, KY 40215
(502) 366-2930
CHIROPRACTIC: Sacro Occipital Technique, Cranial Manipulation, TMJ

LOUISIANA

**DONALD G. KOZAN, D.D.S.**
9886 Hooper Rd.
Baton Rouge, LA 70818-7098
(504) 261-2963
DENTAL: TMJ

**ERNEST WHITMAN, D.C.**
204 E. 69th St.
Shreveport, LA 71106
(318) 861-6311
CHIROPRACTIC: Activator, BEST, Applied Kinesiology, NIMMO

**JOHN SALMON, D.C.**
900 Terry Parkway
New Orleans, LA 70053
(504) 393-2700
CHIROPRACTIC: Applied Kinesiology, COX, Thompson, Physical Therapy, Pettibonn, Activator

**RICHARD HAGES, D.C.**
2614 David Drive
Metairie, LA 70003
(504) 455-4302
CHIROPRACTIC: Palmer, Gonstead, Sacro Occipital Technique, Physical Therapy, Nutrition, Applied Kinesiology, Personal Injury

**WAYNE CRITCHFIELD, D.C.**
6617 Airline Highway
Metairie, LA 70003
(504) 455-6711
CHIROPRACTIC: Full Spine, Applied Kinesiology, Sacro Occipital Technique, Activator, Nutrition, Physical Therapy, Acupressure

**SHERWOOD BEATTY, D.C.**
4141 Veterans Mem. Blvd.
Metairie, LA 70002
(504) 455-2242
CHIROPRACTIC: Full Spine, Applied Kinesiology, Nutrition, Orthopedist, Physical Therapy

**LYLE McFADDEN, D.C.**
P.O. Box 116
Livingston, LA 70754
(504) 686-2292
CHIROPRACTIC: Activator, NIMMO, Diversified, Applied Kinesiology, Sacro Occipital Technique

**ERWIN BIXENMAN, D.C.**
514 N. Antoine St.
Lafayette, LA 70501
(318) 234-4987
CHIROPRACTIC: HIO, PST, Thompson, Cranial, Sacro Occipital Technique, Activator, Chiro. Therapy Adjuncts, Extremities, F.SP.

## MASSACHUSETTES

**GEORGE ATKINS, D.M.D.**
280 Independence Drive
Chestnut Hill
Boston, MA 02167
(617) 327-5777
DENTAL:   TMJ, Cranio-Facial Pain

**GERALD J. MAHER, D.M.D.**
Eye Health Professional Bldg.
696 Main St.
South Weymouth, MA 02190
(617) 337-6644
DENTAL:   TMJ, Cranio-Facial Pain

## MAINE

**JAN ROBERTS, D.C.**
17 Court St.
Farmington, ME 04938
(207) 776-3916
CHIROPRACTIC:   Activator,   Applied
Kinesiology, Nutrition

**ELLEN HOWARD, D.C.**
1570 Broadway
Bangor, ME 04401
(207) 947-3333
CHIROPRACTIC:   Acupuncture, Applied
Kinesiology, Diversified, Nutrition, Physical Therapy, COX, Sacro Occipital Technique, Thompson, Activator

**CHIROPRACTIC   FAMILY   HEALTH
CENTER**
DONALD F. REED, D.C.
17 Third St.
Presque Isle, ME 04769
(207) 764-6595
CHIROPRACTIC:   Nutritional Counsel-
ing (glandular, vitamins and minerals),
Sacro Occipital Technique, Applied Kinesi-
ology, Homeopathy

## MARYLAND

**FULLER MEDICAL CENTER**
MARK LUSTMAN, D.D.S.
6918 Ridge Rd.
Baltimore, MD 21237
(301) 687-4400
DENTAL:   TMJ

**MICHAEL BAYLIN, D.D.S.**
3655 A. Old Court Rd.
Baltimore, MD 21208
(301) 486-6586
DENTAL:   TMJ

**MARK J. McCLURE, D.D.S.**
3500 East West Highway
Hyattsville, MD 20782
(301) 864-5200
DENTAL:   TMJ, General Dentistry

**EDWIN MERRIFIELD, D.C.**
16220 Frederick Ave.
#410
Gaithersburg, MD 20877
(302) 258-8877
CHIROPRACTIC:   Full   Spine,   Applied
Kinesiology, Nutrition, Physical Therapy

**HENRY MILLS, D.C.**
**DIANE ROSSELLO**
6911 Laurel-Bowie Rd.
#206
Bowie, MD 20715
(301) 464-0400
CHIROPRACTIC:   Diversified,   Applied
Kinesiology, Sacro Occipital Technique

**LEWIS CHIROPRACTIC CENTER**
HOWARD F. LEWIS, D.C.
1621-A Belair Rd.
Fallston, MD 21047
(301) 838-2450
(301) 879-3550
CHIROPRACTIC:   Sacro Occipital Technique, Craniopathy, Nutritional Counseling, X-Ray

## MASSACHUSETTS

**DONALD L. BERRY D.M.D.**
332 Washington St. Annex
Wellesley, MA 02181
(617) 235-6900
DENTAL:   TMJ, Functional Oral Orthopedics, Biofeedback, Relaxation Hypnosis,
Stress Management

**JOSHUA KLEEDERMAN, D.C.**
182 Adams Rd.
Williamstown, MA 01267
(413) 458-8102
CHIROPRACTIC:   Sacro Occipital Technique

**KENNETH HARLING, D.C.**
124 Russell St.
Worchester, MA 01609
(617) 753-0503
CHIROPRACTIC:   Applied   Kinesiology,
Palmer, Activator, Gonstead, Diversified

**MARTIN ROSEN, D.C.**
471 Washington St.
Wellesley, MA 02181
(617) 237-6673
CHIROPRACTIC:   Cranial, Sacro Occipital Technique, TMJ, Activator

**DAVID PALOMBO, D.C.**
254 Essex St.
Salem, MA 01970
(617) 744-3590
CHIROPRACTIC:   Applied   Kinesiology,
Activator, Gonstead, Nutrition, Physical
Therapy

**HARMONY CHIROPRACTIC CENTER**
DR. WENDO CARO
DR. RITA L. FIELD
DR. JAN RISING
669 Somerville Ave.
Somerville, MA 02143
(617) 628-9547
CHIROPRACTIC: DNFT, Sacro Occipital Technique, Applied Kinesiology, Cranial, COX, Nutritional Counseling, Physical Therapy

**PAUL HAMILTON, D.C.**
348 Essex St.
Salem, MA 01970
(617) 745-6224
CHIROPRACTIC: Applied Kinesiology, Diversified and Reflex Techniques

**E. QUELLETTE, D.C.**
14 George St.
Norwood, MA 02062
(617) 762-8582
CHIROPRACTIC: Nutrition, Applied Kinesiology, NIMMO, COX, Physical Therapy, Activator, Diversified

**JOHN HAYES, D.C.**
353 Washington St.
Norwell, MA 02061
(617) 659-7989
CHIROPRACTIC: Diversified, Sacro Occipital Technique, COX, Physical Therapy, Nutrition

**ROBERT PROVASOLI, D.C.**
364 Merrimac St.
Newburyport, MA 01950
(617) 465-2311
CHIROPRACTIC: Applied Kinesiology, Sacro Occipital Technique, COX, Nutritional Counseling, Physical Therapy

**THOMAN RUPLEY, D.C.**
120-R School St.
Lexington, MA 02173
(617) 861-6334
CHIROPRACTIC: Diversified, Applied Kinesiology, Activator, Nutrition

**PETER KFOURY, D.C.**
235 Bedford St.
Lexington, MA 02173
(617) 862-7670
CHIROPRACTIC: Thompson, Activator, Applied Kinesiology, Diversified, Sacro Occipital Technique, Nutrition

**BARBARA BECKINGHAM, D.C.**
1137 Main St.
Leominster, MA 01453
(617) 537-8400
CHIROPRACTIC: Activator, Nutrition, Physical Therapy, Gonstead, Sacro Occipital Technique

**JEDD MILLER, D.C.**
39 South St.
Higham, MA 02043
(617) 537-8400
CHIROPRACTIC: Full Spine, Activator, Sacro Occipital Technique, Thompson

**LISA ESPERSON, D.C.**
433 Teaticket Highway
Falmouth, MA 02536
(617) 548-7722
CHIROPRACTIC: Diversified, Activator, Applied Kinesiology, Chiro Manis

**VIVIEN PERGE, D.C.**
2166 Massachusetts Ave.
Cambridge, MA 02140
(617) 492-8300
CHIROPRACTIC: Non-Force Technique, COX, Sacro Occipital Technique, Cranial, Applied Kinesiology

**STEVEN BROWN, D.C.**
129 Mt. Auburn St.
Cambridge, MA 02138
(617) 492-0009
CHIROPRACTIC: Sacro Occipital Technique, Applied Kinesiology, Diversified

**KATHLEEN MEDAGLIA, D.C.**
209 Harvard St.
#500
Brookline, MA 02146
(617) 232-1810
CHIROPRACTIC: Diversified, Applied Kinesiology, Activator, COX, Basic, Physical Therapy, Nutrition, Exercise Evaluation and Program

**MICHELE LAZEROW, D.C.**
1842 Beacon St.
Brookline, MA 02146
(617) 232-8585
CHIROPRACTIC: Activator, Sacro Occipital Technique, Applied Kinesiology, Diversified, Nutrition, Acupuncture

**JAMES DOLAN, D.C.**
1722 Beacon St.
Brookline, MA 02146
(617) 277-2000
CHIROPRACTIC: Pettibon, Grostic, Sacro Occipital Technique, COX

**EDWARD COHEN, D.C.**
1330 Beacon St.
#220
Brookline, MA 02146
(617) 734-7744
CHIROPRACTIC: Sacro Occipital Technique, Motion Palpation, Activator, Diversified

**ANNE LOWEY, D.C.**
**KEN LOWEY, D.C.**
**KEVIN LOWEY, D.C.**
1280 Centre St.
Boston, MA 02159
(617) 332-9080
CHIROPRACTIC: COX, Diversified, Applied Kinesiology, Activator, NIMMO

**TIMOTHY KNIGHT, D.C.**
1122 Massachusetts Ave.
Arlington, MA 02174
(617) 641-2510
CHIROPRACTIC: DNFT, COX, Applied Kinesiology

**THOMAS DEVITA, D.C.**
259 Great Rd.
Acton, MA 01720
(617) 263-9336
CHIROPRACTIC: Sacro Occipital Technique, Activator

**HAMPSHIRE CHIROPRACTIC CENTER**
DAVID M. KOFFMAN, D.C., F.I.C.S.
293 Elm St.
Northampton, MA 01060
(413) 584-7900
CHIROPRACTIC: Nutritional Counseling, Glandular and Natural Vitamins, General Manipulation, Sacro Occipital Technique, Applied Kinesiology

**MICHIGAN**
**JOHN BUCHHEISTER, D.D.S.**
28629 Hoover Rd.
Warren, MI 48093
(313) 751-3950
DENTAL: TMJ, General Dentistry

**LARRY HEARIN, D.D.S.**
2900 E. Grand River Ave.
Howell, MI 48843
(517) 546-7920
DENTAL: TMJ

**ROBERT D. ROUSSEAU, D.D.S.**
**JOHN LIELAIS**
6405 Telegraph Rd.
Bldg. J
Suite 3
Birmingham, MI 48010
(313) 642-5460
DENTAL FUNCTIONAL JAW ORTHOPEDICS: TMJ, Orthodontics/-Orthopedics, Osteopathic Manipulation

**FRANK SALAMONE, D.C.**
810 Biddle Ave.
Wyandotte, MI 48192
(313) 285-4321
CHIROPRACTIC: Kinesiology, Nutrition, Logan Basic, Full Spine

**GARY LORANGER, D.C.**
1811 King Rd.
Trenton, MI 48183
(313) 675-7090
CHIROPRACTIC: COX, Nutrition, Extremities, Full Spine Diversified, Sacro Occipital Technique, Scoliosis, NIMMO, Myotherapy, Barge

**BRUCE FRANKS, D.C.**
1100 S. Carpenter Ave.
Kingsford, MI 49801
(906) 774-3612
CHIROPRACTIC: Palmer, HIO, Gonstead, Applied Kinesiology, Activator

**WAYNE WRIGHT, D.C.**
4301-13 Kalamazoo Ave.
Grand Rapids, MI 49508
(616) 455-7040
CHIROPRACTIC: Full Spine, Applied Kinesiology, Nutrition

**PLAINFIELD CHIROPRACTIC CENTER**
1715 Four Mile Rd., N.E.
Grand Rapids, MI 49505
(616) 363-7771
CHIROPRACTIC: Full Spine Diversified, Sacro Occipital Technique, Applied Kinesiology, Cranial, Gonstead, COX, Nutrition, Physical Therapy, Activator

**GERALD ST. JOHN, D.C.**
3020 Richfield Rd.
Flint, MI 48506
(313) 787-8126
CHIROPRACTIC: Grostic, Palmer Full Spine, COX, Pierce

**5 POINTS CHIROPRACTIC CENTER**
H.R. GRABER, D.C.
19659 US-12 East
Edwardsburg, MI 49112
(616) 641-5520
CHIROPRACTIC: Applied Kinesiology, COX, Activator, Thompson, Full Spine, Nutrition

**JACK SHEREDA, D.C.**
10500 Whittier
Detroit, MI 48224
(313) 526-1810
CHIROPRACTIC: Diversified, Sacro Occipital Technique, COX, Full Spine

**BERNARD MATHEWS, D.C.**
9041 Dexter Blvd.
Detroit, MI 48206
(313) 897-5940
CHIROPRACTIC: Diversified, Applied Kinesiology, Sacro Occipital Technique, Gonstead, Basic, ABCA

**THOMAS LOWREY, D.C.**
19640 Grand River Ave.
Detroit, MI 48223
(313) 531-5113
CHIROPRACTIC: Gonstead, Diversified, Activator, Nutrition, HIO

**MICHAEL KUDIAS, D.C.**
109 Monroe St.
P.O. Box 712
Brooklyn, MI 49230
(517) 592-6180
CHIROPRACTIC: Sacro Occipital Technique, HIO, Stillwagon, Logan Basic

**STEPHEN McCLEAN, D.C.**
1207 Packard
Ann Arbor, MI 48104
(313) 668-6110
CHIROPRACTIC: Sacro Occipital Technique, Cranial, Grostic

**NORMAN EPSTEIN, D.C.**
825 Packard
Ann Arbor, MI 48104
(313) 994-5966
CHIROPRACTIC: Applied Kinesiology, Toftness

**DAVID RUSE, D.C.**
279 Thomas St.
Allegan, MI 49010
(616) 673-5426
CHIROPRACTIC: Sacro Occipital Technique, Palmer Diversified

**WILLIAM McLOUGHLIN, D.C.**
1921 West US 223
Adrian, MI 49221
(517) 263-2900
CHIROPRACTIC: Gonstead, Diversified, Applied Kinesiology

**WARREN H. THOMPSON, D.D.S.**
340 Lovell St. Box 118
Ionia, MI 48846
(616) 527-3050
DENTAL: TMJ, Cranio-Facial Pain

### MINNESOTA

**JOHN WITZIG, D.D.S**
2040 Douglas Drive N.
Minneapolis, MN 55422
(612) 544-0301
DENTAL: TMJ, Dental Orthopedics, Orthodontics, Cranio-Facial Pain

**LESLIE STEWART, D.C.**
1589 Selby Ave.
St. Paul, MN 55104
(612) 644-8242
CHIROPRACTIC: Applied Kinesiology, Diversified, Endocrine, Nutrition

**RICHARD DONAHUE, D.C.**
5 E. County Road B
St. Paul, MN 55117
(612) 488-4043
CHIROPRACTIC: Applied Kinesiology, Activator, Diversified

**CENTER FOR HOLISTIC HEALING**
RUSSELL DESMARIAS, D.C.
569 Selby Ave.
St. Paul, MN 55102
(612) 291-7772
CHIROPRACTIC: Sacro Occipital Technique, Applied Kinesiology, Meridian, Nutrition, Herbs

**DAVID STUSSY, D.C.**
1311 W. 25th St.
Minneapolis, MN 55405
(612) 374-3392
CHIROPRACTIC: Diversified, Activator, Acupuncture, NIMMO, Applied Kinesiology, Spinal Stress, Spinal Touch, Nutrition

**AARONN FLICKSTEIN, D.C.**
3300 Penn Ave. N.
Minneapolis, MN 55412
(612) 529-9605
CHIROPRACTIC: Applied Kinesiology, Nutrition, Herbs, Homeopathy

**TATIANA RIABOKIN, D.C.**
1521 Excelsior Ave. West
Hopkins, MN 55343
(612) 935-9360
CHIROPRACTIC: Applied Kinesiology, Sacro Occipital Technique, Diversified, Acupuncture, Activator, Nutrition

**SKIBTED CHIROPRACTIC OFFICES**
1821 St. Clair Ave.
St. Paul, MN 55105
(612) 699-3366
CHIROPRACTIC: Sacro Occipital Technique, Applied Kinesiology, Craniopathy, TMJ

### MISSISSIPPI

**DONALD HUMBERG, D.C.**
205 W. Northside Drive
Jackson, MS 39206
(601) 366-8300
CHIROPRACTIC: Palmer Diversified, Activator, Sacro Occipital Technique, COX, Spinal Touch

### MISSOURI

**ROBERT RIMMER, D.C.**
2359 Chambers Rd.
St. Louis, MO 63136
(314) 868-2220
CHIROPRACTIC: Meric, Applied Kinesiology, Physical Therapy, Acupuncture, Nutrition

**KENNETH OSIA, D.C.**
5600 S. Compton Ave.
St. Louis, MO 63111
(314) 351-6308
CHIROPRACTIC: Diversified, Sacro Occipital Technique, Basic, Gonstead, Applied Kinesiology, Nutrition

**JILL FRANK, D.C.**
10455 Old Olive St.
St. Louis, MO 63141
(314) 569-2640
CHIROPRACTIC: Diversified, NIMMO, Applied Kinesiology, Physical Therapy

**DARRELL BLAIN, D.C.**
77 Charleston Square
St. Charles, MO 63303
(314) 441-5600
CHIROPRACTIC: Pierce Stillwagon, COX, Applied Kinesiology

**JOHN T. HADDER, D.C.**
1320 S. Glenstone
Suite 12-A
Springfield, MO 65804
(417) 883-1141
CHIROPRACTIC: Sacro Occipital Technique, Cranial Manipulation, TMJ, Nutritional Counseling, Nutritional Therapy

**SYLVIA BARTLETT, D.C.**
**BEVERLY MILES**
Edgar Star Route
Box 207
Rolla, MO 65401
(314) 364-3919
CHIROPRACTIC: Sacro Occipital Technique, Cranial, Activator, STO, Nutrition

**JOHN NOLAN, D.C.**
121 S. Kansas Ave.
Marceline, MO 64658
(816) 376-3331
CHIROPRACTIC: Activator, Applied Kinesiology, Basic, Nutrition, Meridian Therapy, Physical Therapy

**KIM CARRAHER, D.C.**
1007-B Southwest Blvd.
Jefferson City, MO 65101
(314) 634-5155
CHIROPRACTIC: Applied Kinesiology, Logan Basic, Diversified, Nutrition

**DALE JOHNSON, D.C.**
14 E. 20th St.
Higginsville, MO 64037
(816) 584-2338
CHIROPRACTIC: Applied Kinesiology, Full Spine, Activator, Nutrition

**DANA ROBERTSON, D.C.**
711-C Vandiver Drive
Columbia, MO 65202
(314) 874-3365
CHIROPRACTIC: Diversified, Basic, Best, Extremity, Nutrition, Adjunctive therapy, Sacro Occipital Technique

**GEORGE HECHLER, D.C.**
635 S. Main
Brookfield, MO 64628
(816) 258-2236
CHIROPRACTIC: Meridan Therapy, Activator, Applied Kinesiology, Nutrition, Physical Therapy

**MARCY ALLEN GOLDSTEIN, M.D.**
950 Francis Pl.
Suite 301
Clayton, MO 63105
(314) 725-9105
MEDICAL: Acupuncture

**SHEALY PAIN AND HEALTH REHABILITATION INSTITUTE**
C. NORMAN SHEALY, M.D., Ph.D.
3525 S. National
Suite 207
Springfield, MO 65807
(417) 882-0850
MEDICAL, STRESS MANAGEMENT, PREVENTIVE MEDICINE: Nutritional Counseling, Osteopathic Manipulation, Acupuncture, Transcutaneous Electrical Nerve Stimulation, Biofeedback, Self-Regulation Training, Psychological Counseling

**ATRIUM HEALTH SERVICES**
JOSEPH F. UNGER, JR., D.C.
4224 Watson Rd.
St. Louis, MO 63109
(314) 352-7233
CHIROPRACTIC: SOT, Cranial, Classical Homeopathy

**DELCREST CHIROPRACTIC**
DAVID L. ROZEBOOM, D.C.
8428 Delmar
St. Louis, MO 63124
(314) 997-2308
CHIROPRACTIC: Sacro Occipital Technique, Applied Kinesiology, Nutritional Counseling, Thermography, Live Cell Analysis

## MONTANA

**OLD CHURCH CHIROPRACTIC CENTER**
DRS. ROBERT and RUTH ANN HAGER, D.C.
505 Fourth Ave. W.
Columbia Falls, MT 59912
(406) 892-4331
CHIROPRACTIC: Applied Kinesiology, Gonstead, Diversified, Sacro Occipital Technique, Nutrition

**PLAZA WEST DENTAL GROUP**
1537 Ave. D
Billings, MT 59102
(406) 248-7171
DENTAL: TMJ Dysfunction, Cranio-Facial Pain, General Dentistry

## NEBRASKA

**EDGAR POSSIN, D.C.**
5011 Grover St.
Omaha, NE 681-6
(402) 551-6333
CHIROPRACTIC: Sacro Occipital Technique, Activator, Physical Therapy

**CASEY IVERSON, D.C.**
702 W. Koenig
Grand Island, NE 68801
(308) 382-3666
CHIROPRACTIC: Applied Kinesiology, COX, Activator, Nutrition, Laser Acupuncture, Diversified, Physical Therapy

**MAJOR B. DeJARNETTE, D.O, D.C.**
722 1/2 Central Ave.
Nebraska City, NE 68410
(402) 873-6769
CHIROPRACTIC: Sacro Occipital Technique, Cranial Manipulation

## NEVADA

**REID BRECKE, D.C.**
33 St. Lawrence
Reno, NV 89509
(702) 329-5950
CHIROPRACTIC: NUCCA, PST, NVD, Sacro Occipital Technique

**MARK BAXTER, D.C.**
3421 E. Tropicanna #G
Las Vegas, NV 89121
(702) 451-0461
CHIROPRACTIC: Gonstead, Applied Kinesiology, Nutrition

**GREEN VALLEY CHIROPRACTIC**
CRAIG ROLES, D.C.
2720 Green Valley Parkway
Henderson, NV 89015
(702) 451-0480
CHIROPRACTIC: Motion Palpation, Applied Kinesiology, COX, Nutrition, Diversified

## NEW HAMPSHIRE

**JOHN B. KENISON, D.D.S.**
45 Amherst St.
Milford, NH 03055
(603) 673-1233
DENTAL: TMJ

**GERALD PEARCE, D.C.**
24 Washington St.
Exeter, NH 03833
(603) 772-5631
CHIROPRACTIC: Gonstead, Applied Kinesiology, COX, Physical Therapy

**WELLSPRING CHIROPRACTIC HEALTH CENTER**
DRS. TERRY R. HORWITZ and JOEL S. SHRUT, D.C.
8 Hanson St.
Dover, NH 03820
(603) 742-3270
CHIROPRACTIC: Diversified, Sacro Occipital Technique, Activator, COX, Nutrition

## NEW JERSEY

**IRA M. KLEMONS, D.D.S., Ph.D.**
499 Ernston Rd.
Parlin, NJ 08859
(201) 727-5000
DENTAL: TMJ, Cranio-Facial Pain

**WILLIAM V. CIRINO, JR., D.C.**
514 Lafayette Ave.
Hawthorne, NJ 07506
(201) 427-6663
CHIROPRACTIC: Sacro Occipital Technique, Cranial Manipulation, Nutritional Counseling

**ROBERT MONOKIAN, D.C.**
1201 W. Marlton Pike
Cherry Hill, NJ 08034
(609) 428-5756
CHIROPRACTIC: Applied Kinesiology, Cranial Manipulation, Sports Injuries, Nutritional Counseling, Acuscope Scope, Acupressure

**ALAN WENDER, D.D.S.**
362 Ridgeway
Mt. Holly, NJ 08060
(609) 267-3230
DENTAL: TMJ, Cranio-Facial Pain, Cranial Manipulation, Nutritional Counseling, Dental Orthopedics, General Dentistry, Mercury Free Fillings

**JOEL ISERSON, D.D.S.**
TWIN RIVERS PROFESSIONAL BLDG.
Route 33
East Windsor, NJ 08520
(609) 443-1112
DENTAL: TMJ

**SAM ZIMMERMAN, D.C.**
196 Broad St.
Red Bank, NJ 07701
(201) 842-3302
CHIROPRACTIC: Sacro Occipital Technique

**HARVEY GETZOFF, D.C.**
**STEPHEN LESSE**
11 W. Main St.
Marlton, NJ 08053
(609) 983-0009
CHIROPRACTIC: Sacro Occipital Technique, Craniopathy, TMJ, Nutritional Counseling, Diversified

**CATHERINE SPEARS, M.D.**
25 Red Rd.
Chatham, NJ 07928
(201) 635-8795
NEUROLOGY: Acupuncture, Neurology

**JAMES TIGHE, D.C.**
630 Salem Pike
Woodbury, NJ 08096
(609) 853-7577
CHIROPRACTIC: Diversified, Sacro Occipital Technique, Applied Kinesiology, COX, Physical Therapy, Thompson, Pierce

**PETER BOULUKIOS, D.C.**
175 Cedar Lane
Teaneck, NJ 07666
(201) 836-2838
CHIROPRACTIC: Sacro Occipital Technique, DNFT, Applied Kinesiology, Activator, Nutrition, Soft Tissue

**SPARTA FAMILY CHIROPRACTIC CENTER**
WILLIAM DEGASPERIS, D.C.
CHRISTOPHER BUMP, D.C.
270 Sparta Ave. #209
Sparta, NJ 07871
(201) 729-8680
CHIROPRACTIC: Applied Kinesiology, Sacro Occipital Technique, Cranial, COX, TMJ, Nutrition, Activator, Physical Therapy

**FRED KINGSBURY, D.C.**
764 Easton Ave.
Somerset, NJ 08873
(201) 247-1020
CHIROPRACTIC: Applied Kinesiology, Chiromanis, Sacro Occipital Technique, Logan, NIMMO, Nutrition, Inversion Gravity System, Cert. Team Physician

**DAVID KUTSCHMAN, D.C.**
**DANIEL KUTSCHMAN, D.C.**
682 Broad St.
Shrewsbury, NJ 07701
(201) 530-4077
CHIROPRACTIC: Applied Kinesiology, Activator, Chiromanis, Full Spine, Physiotherapy, Nutrition, PST

**JAMES DUBEL, D.C.**
225 Highway 35
Red Bank, NJ 07701
(201) 747-4646
CHIROPRACTIC: Multi D.C. Practice, Diversified, Gonstead, Sacro Occipital Technique

**MICHAEL D. WARNER, D.C.**
2124 Bridge Ave.
Point Pleasant, NJ 08742
(201) 892-5775
CHIROPRACTIC: Diversified, Full Spine, Activator, Sacro Occipital Technique

**BOOS CHIROPRACTIC CENTER**
PHILIP H. BOOS, D.C.
2 Frederick St.
Morristown, NJ 07960
(201) 539-8877
CHIROPRACTIC: Palmer Diversified, Thompson, Logan, Sacro Occipital Technique, Physical Therapy

**DRS. URCIUOLI, BALON, MAZANOWSKI**
289 Central Ave.
Metuchen, NJ 08840
(201) 549-0141
CHIROPRACTIC: Diversified, Sacro Occipital Technique, Applied Kinesiology, Activator

**KAREN ROBINSON, D.C.**
440 Ridge Rd.
Lyndhurst, NJ 07071
(201) 460-9010
CHIROPRACTIC: Applied Kinesiology, Nutritional Counseling, Physiotherapy

**EARLE BRYAN, D.C.**
38 Smith St.
Irvington, NJ 07111
(201) 374-3868
CHIROPRACTIC: Diversified, Kinesiology

## RICHARD SANTUCCI, D.C.
547 Main St.
Hackensack, NJ 07601
(201) 343-8282
CHIROPRACTIC: COX, Thompson, HIO, Sacro Occipital Technique, Activator

## GENE PATERNO, D.C.
192 Prospect Ave.
Hackensack, NJ 07601
(201) 342-5585
CHIROPRACTIC: Diversified, Sacro Occipital Technique, Sports, Therapy, Applied Kinesiology

## CHARLES CALABRESE, D.C.
210 Spring Valley Ave.
Hackensack, NJ 07601
(201) 342-8002
CHIROPRACTIC: Diversified, Sacro Occipital Technique, Applied Kinesiology, Thompson, Sports Injuries, Activator, Nutrition

## PAUL FRANZ, D.C.
570 Mountain Ave.
Gillette, NJ 07933
(201) 647-5200
CHIROPRACTIC: Applied Kinesiology, Full Spine, HIO, PST, Logan, Gonstead

## CHARLES FERRANTE, D.C.
71 W. Main St.
Freehold, NJ 07728
(201) 780-6550
CHIROPRACTIC: COX, Full Spine, Sacro Occipital Technique

## ELLIOT KOZIEL, D.C.
1625 Lemoine Ave.
Fort Lee, NJ 07024
(201) 592-1378
CHIROPRACTIC: Applied Kinesiology, Sacro Occipital Technique, Diversified, Activator

## STE HEN PRESS, D.C.
546 Broad Ave.
Englewood, NJ 07631
(201) 569-1444
CHIROPRACTIC: Diversified, Applied Kinesiology, Sacro Occipital Technique, Logan, Physical Therapy

## KENNETH FREEDMAN, D.C.
Brier Hill Court D-6
East Brunswick, NJ 08816
(201) 254-6011
CHIROPRACTIC: HIO Specific, Full Spine, Sacro Occipital Technique, Thompson

## WULSTER, JERSEY and TERRY, D.C.
35 W. Main St.
#206
Denville, NJ 07834
(201) 627-6980
CHIROPRACTIC: MPI, Diversified, Applied Kinesiology, Nutrition, Activator

## ART KELLENBERGER, D.C.
44 Leigh St.
Clinton, NJ 08809
(201) 735-4086
CHIROPRACTIC: PST, Diversified, Applied Kinesiology, Sacro Occipital Technique, Physical Therapy, Logan, COX

## JEFFREY HORNING, D.C.
116 W. Broad St.
Burlington, NJ 08016
(609) 387-4166
CHIROPRACTIC: Applied Kinesiology, Sacro Occipital Technique, COX, Full Spine, Nutrition

## ALBERT CHINAPPI, D.D.S
43 E. Main St.
Marlton, NJ 08053
(609) 983-5559
DENTAL: Orthodontics, Dental Orthopedics, TMJ

## DAVID CHEETHAM, D.C.
505 Station Ave.
Haddon Heights, NJ 08035
(609) 547-2965
CHIROPRACTIC: Applied Kinesiology, Cranial Manipulation, TMJ, Nutritional Counseling

## RICHARD R. COBB, D.C.
207 Haddon Ave.
Haddonfield, NJ 08033
(609) 429-4464
CHIROPRACTIC: Applied Kinesiology, Thermography, Sacro Occipital Technique, TMJ, Craniopathy

## ROBERT S. FISHER, D.C.
8 Main St.
P.O. Box 702
Flemington, NJ 08822
(201) 788-1714
CHIROPRACTIC: Physical Therapy, Activator Technique, Diversified Technique, Logan Basic

## PRINCETON BRAIN BIO CENTER
CARL C. PFEIFFER, M.D.
862 Route 518
Skillman, NJ 08558-0025
(609) 924-8607
MEDICAL: Allergy Unit, Amino Acid Testing, Orthomolecular Medicine, Nutrition Counseling

**JAMES SPINELLI, D.D.S.**
5924 Westfield Ave.
Pennsauken, NJ 08110
(609) 663-4881
DENTAL: Orthodontics, Dental Orthopedics, TMJ

**ROCKAWAY CHIROPRACTIC CENTER**
DR. PAUL B. BINDELL
75 East Main St.
Rockaway, NJ 07866
(201) 625-0500
CHIROPRACTIC: Applied     Kinesiology,
Nutrition

## NEW MEXICO

**JOHN D. ARNOLD, D.C.**
3737 Eubank Blvd. N.E.
Albuquerque, NM 87111
(505) 266-3441
CHIROPRACTIC: Sacro     Occipital     Technique, Craniopathy, TMJ

**ERVIN DAILEY, D.C.**
P.O. Box 1800
Farmington, N.M.  87499
(505) 325-7784
CHIROPRACTIC: Sacro     Occipital     Technique, Lower Back Pain, TMJ

**NOREEN SULLIVAN, D.C.**
1301 Luisa St.
Santa Fe, NM 87501
(505) 982-0691
CHIROPRACTIC: Applied     Kinesiology,
GEA, Nutrition, Allergy, Sacro Occipital
Technique, Cranial, Athletics

**DARRELL ATCHLEY, D.C.**
1601 W. Ave. 1
Lovington, NM 88260
(505) 396-5307
CHIROPRACTIC: HIO, Pettibon, Thompson, Applied Kinesiology, De Jarnette

**GUILLERMO GRADILLAS, D.C.**
1111 E. Lohman Ave.
Las Cruces, NM 88001
(505) 523-7594
CHIROPRACTIC: DNFT, Applied Kinesiology, Electro Acupuncture, Meric, Physical Therapy

**LAWRENCE GREGORY, D.C.**
3001 N. Prince
Clovis, NM 88101
(505) 763-6948
CHIROPRACTIC: Toftness, Sacro Occipital Technique, Cranial, Activator, Gonstead

**CIVIC     CENTER     CHIROPRACTIC OFFICES**
ERVIN R. DAILEY, D.C.
312 W. La Plata St.
P.O. Box 1800
Farmington, NM 87499
(505) 326-1995
CHIROPRACTIC: Nutritional Counseling, Craniopathy, Sacro Occipital Technique, Chiropractic Orthopedics, Hypnotherapy

## NEW YORK

**TENTH STREET CHIROPRACTIC**
MICHAEL CINDRICH, D.C.
15 E. 10th St. 1-C
New York, NY 10003
(212) 982-4449
CHIROPRACTIC: TMJ, Sacro Occipital Technique, Applied Kinesiology, Nutritional Counseling, Cranial Manipulation, Sports Injuries

**SANDY HOLLOW CHIROPRACTIC OFFICE**
DEBORAH KLEINMAN-CINDRICH, D.C.
33 Sandy Hollow Rd.
Port Washington, NY 11050
(516) 883-1305
CHIROPRACTIC: TMJ, Sacro Occipital Technique, Applied Kinesiology, Nutritional Counseling, Cranial Manipulation, Sports Injuries

**DR. JOHN G. RUPOLO**
148 Tulip Ave.
Floral Park, NY 11001
(516) 354-4310
CHIROPRACTIC: Sacro Occipital Technique, Applied Kinesiology, Acupressure, Nutritional     Counseling,     Homeopathy, Physiotherapy, Brain Wave Reduplication, Craniofacial Stabilizers

**HAROLD GELB, D.M.D.**
635 Madison Ave.
New York, NY 10022
(212) 752-1661
DENTAL: TMJ, Head, Neck and Facial Pain, Nutritional Counseling

**MICHAEL R. MARFINO, D.D.S.**
5893 Main St.
Williamsville, NY 14221
(716) 631-3322
DENTAL: TMJ

**LAWRENCE DE MANN, D.C.**
300 E. 56th
New York City, NY 10022
(212) 688-2016
CHIROPRACTIC: Sacro Occipital Technique, Craniopathy, TMJ, Diversified

**JOHN DACCARDI, D.C.**
263 New Rt.
Stony Point, NY 10980
(914) 942-0256
CHIROPRACTIC: Activator, Applied
Kinesiology, Gonstead

**MARIO INTRONA, D.C.**
3930 Richmond Ave.
Staten Island, NY 10312
(718) 356-5560
CHIROPRACTIC: HIO, Applied Kinesiology,
Sacro Occipital Technique, TMJ, Chiromanis, Nutrition, Activator, Trigger,
Physical Therapy

**LOUIS LUPINACCI, D.C.**
555 Lake Ave.
St. James, NY 11780
(516) 862-6207
CHIROPRACTIC: Diversified, Sacro Occipital Technique, COX, Physical Therapy,
Nutrition

**JUDSON WERBELA, D.C.**
2599 Elmwood Ave.
Rochester, NY 14609
(716) 288-7800
CHIROPRACTIC: Diversified, Applied
Kinesiology, Acupressure, Nutrition, COX

**DONALD SEIDEL, D.C.**
972 Culver Rd.
Rochester, NY 14609
(716) 288-7800
CHIROPRACTIC: Gonstead, Applied Kinesiology, Sacro Occipital Technique

**DAVID REICH, D.C.**
86-04 117 St.
Richmond Hill, NY 11418
(718) 847-5252
CHIROPRACTIC: Diversified Full Spine,
COX, Sacro Occipital Technique, Applied
Kinesiology, TMJ

**MARK HEFFRON, D.C.**
80-03 211th St.
Hollis Hills, Queens, NY 11427
(212) 464-8948
CHIROPRACTIC: Activator, Diversified,
Zindler, Sacro Occipital Technique, Physical Therapy

**GLEN NYKWEST, D.C.**
503 Bedford Rd.
Pleasantville, NY 10570
(914) 769-6007
CHIROPRACTIC: Diversified, Applied
Kinesiology, Physical Therapy, Nutrition

**GREGORY GUMBERICH, D.C.**
208 Guinea Woods Rd.
Old Westbury, NY 11568
(516) 294-9494
CHIROPRACTIC: COX, Applied Kinesiology, HIO, Gonstead, Physical Therapy,
Nutrition, Sacro Occipital Technique

**MICHAEL WOLFF, D.C.**
300 E. 57th St.
New York City, NY 10022
(212) 688-3704
CHIROPRACTIC: Applied Kinesiology,
Sacro Occipital Technique, Activator,
Diversified, Nutrition

**JOSEPH MIRTO, D.C.**
580 Park Ave.
New York City, NY 10021
(212) 838-6600
CHIROPRACTIC: Applied Kinesiology,
Sacro Occipital Technique, Cranial, Harmonics, Nutritional Counseling

**STEVEN M. PERMAN, D.C.**
1101 Jericho Turnpike
New Hyde Park, NY 11040
(516) 328-3322
CHIROPRACTIC: Applied Kinesiology,
Cranial Adjustments, TMJ, Sports Injuries,
Wholistic Health Center

**NANCY JACOBS, D.C.**
67 Park Ave.
New York City, NY 10016
(212) 696-4444
CHIROPRACTIC: Diversified, Sacro Occipital Technique, HIO, Activator, Nutrition,
Physical Therapy

**MICHAEL CINDRICH, D.C.**
14 W. Ninth St.
New York City, NY 10011
(212) 982-4449
CHIROPRACTIC: Sacro Occipital Technique, Applied Kinesiology, Nutrition,
Cranial, Receptor Tonus

**HAROLD ORR, D.C.**
516 Lakeville Rd.
New Hyde Park, NY 11040
(516) 775-0778
CHIROPRACTIC: Gonstead, COX, Applied
Kinesiology, Physical Therapy

**EVAN LADOUX, D.C.**
944 Park Ave.
Manhattan, NY 10028
(212) 628-5353
CHIROPRACTIC: F.SP, HIO, COX, Applied
Kinesiology, Perry, Activator, Extremity,
Physical Therapy, ACU SLP, MYO PLS

**SCOTT SIMERMAN, D.C.**
516 W. Boston Post Rd.
Mamaroneck, NY 10543
(914) 381-4777
CHIROPRACTIC: Activator, Applied Kinesiology, HIO, Sacro Occipital Technique, Diversified Full Spine

**DRS. EISMAN and GRUSHACK, D.C.**
714 E. Park Ave.
Long Beach, NY 11561
(516) 431-7972
CHIROPRACTIC: Sacro Occipital Technique, Applied Kinesiology, Diversified, Nutrition, COX

**MICHELE COHEN, D.C.**
429 E. Park Ave.
Long Beach, NY 11561
(516) 432-7300
CHIROPRACTIC: Activator, Diversified, Applied Kinesiology

**HENRY COHEN, D.C.**
133 Larchmont Ave.
Larchmont, NY 10538
(914) 834-1606
CHIROPRACTIC: Applied Kinesiology, Sacro Occipital Technique, Diversified, COX, Activator, Nutrition

**RONALD GOODMARK, D.C.**
199 Oakwood Rd.
Huntington, NY 11743
(516) 271-5188
CHIROPRACTIC: Pettibon, Sacro Occipital Technique, Cranial, Activator, Diversified

**ALAN FURMAN, D.C.**
199 Oakwood Rd.
Huntington, NY 11743
(516) 271-7770
CHIROPRACTIC: Pettibon, Diversified, Sacro Occipital Technique, Activator

**KEITH NELSON, D.C.**
58 Broadway
Greenlawn, NY 11740
(516) 754-1666
CHIROPRACTIC: Gonstead, Full Spine, Sacro Occipital Technique, COX

**MATTHEW MARGRAF, D.C.**
32-32 Francis Lewis Blvd.
Flushing, NY 11358
(718) 762-3811
CHIROPRACTIC: Full Spine, Diversified, Applied Kinesiology, Sacro Occipital Technique

**ALLEN CHIROPRACTIC HOLISTIC HEALTH CARE CENTER**
GIL ALLEN, D.C.
142-01 37th Ave.
Flushing, NY 11354
(212) 461-7788
CHIROPRACTIC: Diversified, Applied Kinesiology, Sacro Occipital Technique, Reflexology, Nutrition, COX

**JAMES VANDENBERG, D.C.**
140 E. Elm St.
East Rochester, NY 14445
(716) 586-4785
CHIROPRACTIC: Full Spine, Activator, Applied Kinesiology

**EUGENE HALLER, D.C.**
34 Fieldview Lane
East Hampton, NY 11937
(516) 324-1037
CHIROPRACTIC: Thompson, Activator, Applied Kinesiology, Sacro Occipital Technique, Diversified

**BARRY COHEN, D.C.**
357 E. Main St.
Centerport, NY 11721
(516) 673-3300
CHIROPRACTIC: Diversified Full Spine, Chiromanis, Logan, HIO, Pierce Stillwagon, Cranial, Sacro Occipital Technique

**THOMAS WRIGHT, D.C.**
470 S. Pearl St.
Canadaigua, NY 14424
(716) 394-2030
CHIROPRACTIC: Applied Kinesiology, Cranial, Activator, Logan Basic, Sacro Occipital Technique

**ANTHONY MAGNANO, D.C.**
2477 Union Rd.
Buffalo, NY 14227
(716) 668-5553
CHIROPRACTIC: HIO, Full Spine, Thompson, Gonstead, Sacro Occipital Technique, Diversified, Extremity, Chiromanis, Nutrition

**CHARLES LOWE, D.C.**
519 Lefferts Ave.
Brooklyn, NY 11225
(212) 493-9201
CHIROPRACTIC: All Chiropractic Techniques

**MAUREEN MOORE, D.C.**
489 Throgs Neck Expressway
Bronx, NY 10465
(212) 863-0072
CHIROPRACTIC: Applied Kinesiology, Full Spine Diversified, Sacro Occipital Technique, COX, Nutritional and Physiotherapy Available

**OERZEN CHIROPRACTIC ASSOCIATION**
248-36 Jericho Turnpike
Bellerose, NY 11001
(516) 352-7111
CHIROPRACTIC: Straight, Palmer (HIO),
Sacro Occipital Technique, Diversified

**MYLES O'REILLY, D.C.**
2581 W. End Ave.
Baldwin, NY 11510
(516) 868-7777
CHIROPRACTIC: Activator, DNFT, Applied
Kinesiology, Sacro Occipital Technique

**ARTHUR KRIEGER, D.C.**
38-04 Thirty-first Ave.
Astoria, NY 11103
(212) 726-0404
CHIROPRACTIC: Sacro Occipital Technique, Full Spine

**CARL MESTMAN, D.D.S.**
226 7th St., Suite 305
Garden City, NY 11530
(914) 561-4804
DENTAL: TMJ, Dental Orthopedics, Cranial Manipulation, Sacro Occipital Technique, Nutritional Counseling, Acupuncture, Toxicology (Removal of Mercury Fillings), Reflexology

**THOMAS ROGOWSKEY, D.C.**
55 W. 90th St. #3
New York, NY 10024
(212) 362-1733
CHIROPRACTIC: Applied Kinesiology,
Directed Non-Force Technique, Nutritional
Counseling

**MOUNTAINVIEW MEDICAL ASSOCIATES**
NEIL BLOCK, M.D.
MICHAEL SCHACHTER, M.D.
Mountainview Ave.
Nyack, NY 10960
(914) 358-6800
MEDICAL: Holistic Approach (Traditional
and Alternative Care), Nutritional Counseling, Orthomolecular Psychiatry and
Medicine, Chelation Therapy, Environmental Medicine (Clinical Ecology) and
Allergies, Colonics, Acupuncture

**DR. RONALD R. BLAND**
BROADWAY CHIROPRACTIC CENTER
230 W. 55th St.
New York, NY 10019
(212) 246-2330
CHIROPRACTIC: Applied Kinesiology,
Sacro Occipital Technique, Nutritional
Healing, Manipulative Therapy, Hair
Analysis, Sports Injuries

**NORTH CAROLINA**

**RICHARD LEWIS, D.C.**
5107 Ralls of the Neuse
Raleigh, NC 27609
(919) 878-0111
CHIROPRACTIC: COX, Motion Palpation,
Applied Kinesiology

**TUNIS HUNT, D.C.**
5401 S. Blvd.
Charlotte, NC 28210
(704) 523-7454
CHIROPRACTIC: Activator, PST, Kinesiology, Diversified

**GARY FARR, D.C.**
1401-H E. Maynard Rd.
Cary, NC 27511
(919) 467-7187
CHIROPRACTIC: Activator, COX, Applied
Kinesiology, Nutrition, Physical Therapy,
Acupuncture

**MURRAY GREENSPAN, D.C.**
Rt. 70
P.O. Box 145
Black Mountain, NC 28711
(704) 686-3873
CHIROPRACTIC: Applied Kinesiology,
COX, Physiotherapy

**CALLOWAY CHIROPRACTIC CLINIC**
JOHN V.N. BANDY, D.C.
Sunset Dr.
P.O. Box 467
Blowing Rock, NC 28605
(204) 295-9896
CHIROPRACTIC: Applied Kinesiology,
SOT, Homeopathy, Nutrition, Herbs

**WALTER H. SCHMITT, JR., D.C.**
87 S. Elliott Rd.
Suite 110
Chapel Hill, NC 27514
(919) 942-8516
CHIROPRACTIC: Applied Kinesiology,
Cranial Manipulation, Nutritional Counseling, TMJ

**NORTH DAKOTA**

**ARNOLD SIEFKEN, D.C.**
Jamestown Mall #215
Jamestown, ND 58401
(701) 252-0569
CHIROPRACTIC: Applied Kinesiology,
Activator, Full Spine Diversified, Physical
Therapy

**VALLEY WEST HEALTH CENTER OR
THOMSEN CHIROPRACTIC CLINIC**
DR. KIM B. FOELL, D.C.
DR. ROBERT L. THOMSEN, D.C.
Box 447 W. Main
Valley City, ND 58072
(701) 845-2481
CHIROPRACTIC: Nutritional Counseling,
Natural Vitamins, Applied Kinesiology,
Acupuncture

# OHIO

**LEE W. STAHL, D.D.S.**
1558 S. Byrne #B
Toledo, OH 43614
(419) 693-2024
DENTAL: Dental Orthopedics, Orthodontics, TMJ

**CHIROPRACTIC HEALTH CLINIC**
DR. JAMES T. SCHMIT
806 E. Wayne Street
Celina, OH 45822
(419) 586-7776
CHIROPRACTIC: Sacro Occipital Technique, Nutritional Counseling and Testing,
Allergy Testing, Homeopathy, Neurological
Organization Technique, Learning Disabilities and Dyslexia

**DR. PHILIP C. ROBBINS**
Route 5, Box 221B
Pleasant Hill Rd.
Athens, OH 45701
(614) 593-6333
OSTEOPATHIC: General Medicine, Homeopathy, Nutritional Counseling

**STEPHEN V. LEE, D.D.S**
3140 Dayton-Xenia Rd.
Beavercreek, OH 45385
(513) 426-4024
DENTAL: General Dentistry, TMJ

**T.G. LEATHERMAN, D.D.S**
6111 S. Broadway
Lorain, OH 44053
(216) 233-8521
DENTAL: TMJ, General Dentistry

**ROBERT WOLLENSCHLAGER, D.C.**
1916 N. Reynolds Rd.
Toledo, OH 43615
(419) 536-5446
CHIROPRACTIC: Applied Kinesiology,
Diversified

**CATHERINE NUNIER, D.C.
DANIEL LYNCH, D.C.**
2177 Olympic
Springfield, OH 45503
(513) 390-6138
CHIROPRACTIC: Diversified, Sacro
Occipital Technique, Basic, Nutrition,
Physical Therapy

**ROBERT FORBES, D.C.**
50 Liberty St. Extension
Painesville, OH 44077
(216) 357-6200
CHIROPRACTIC: Activator, Applied Kinesiology, PCRF

**MICHAEL KLOSTERMAN, D.C.**
931 Highway 28
Milford, OH 45150
(513) 831-0830
CHIROPRACTIC: Applied Kinesiology,
Diversified, Activator, Nutrition

**DAVID POLEN, D.C.**
2675 Medway New Carlisle Rd.
Medway, OH 45341
(513) 849-1349
CHIROPRACTIC: Sacro Occipital Technique, Cranial, Nutrition

**JOSEPH ANDREJCIK, D.C.**
908 W. Main St.
Louisville, OH 44641
(216) 875-3400
CHIROPRACTIC: Specific and General
Techniques, Applied Kinesiology, Modalities

**ARTHUR HOLMES, D.C.**
111 W. Walnut St.
Hillsboro, OH 45133
(513) 393-2313
CHIROPRACTIC: Diplomate of Applied
Kinesiology, COX, Diversified, Deimbrication, Physical Therapy, Nutrition

**PAUL SILER, D.C.**
910 Downs St.
Defiance, OH 43512
(419) 782-0956
CHIROPRACTIC: Palmer Diversified,
Gonstead, Applied Kinesiology

**THOMAS KREUSCH, D.C.**
3821 Little York Rd.
Dayton/Vandalia, OH 45414
(513) 898-7023
CHIROPRACTIC: Grostic, Gonstead, COX,
Sacro Occipital Technique, Applied Kinesiology, Spinal Stressology

**MIKEL and PATRICIA LYDY, D.C.**
Rt. 2
County Line Rd.
Crestline, OH 44827
(419) 683-1298
CHIROPRACTIC: Sacro Occipital Technique, Grostic, COX, Diversified, Nutrition

**CYNTHIA ZARTMAN, D.C.**
912 King Ave.
Columbus, OH 43212
(614) 291-2029
CHIROPRACTIC: Diversified, COX, Applied Kinesiology, Basic, Physical Therapy,
Activator, BTHAA

**HAROLD KENNEY, D.C.**
572 N. Main St.
Akron, OH 44310
(216) 376-7587
CHIROPRACTIC: Orthopedics, COX Procedures, Craniopathy, Sacro Occipital Technique, Physiological Therapeutics

**SYLVANIA HEALTH CLINIC**
DAVID M. DIPAOLO, D.C.
4930 Holland-Sylvania Rd.
Sylvania, OH 43560
(419) 882-7148
CHIROPRACTIC: Nutritional Counseling, Acupressure, Applied Kinesiology, Natuopathy, Macrobiotic Counseling, Massage Therapy, Intermittant Spinal Traction

**DANIEL H. DUFFY, D.C.**
299 S. Broadway
Geneva, OH 44041
(216) 466-1186
CHIROPRACTIC: Applied Kinesiology, Cranial Manipulation, Nutritional Counseling, TMJ

## OKLAHOMA

**CHARLES TUCKER, D.D.S.**
Box 388
Alva, OK 73717
(405) 327-2277
DENTAL: TMJ

**ROBERT BUTTS, D.C.**
1217-C S. 11th St.
Yukon, OK 73099
(405) 354-5231
CHIROPRACTIC: Applied Kinesiology, Diversified, Sacro Occipital Technique, Gonstead, Physical Therapy

**R.E. PARKER, D.C.**
12929 E. 21st St.
#G
Tulsa, OK 74134
(918) 438-2377
CHIROPRACTIC: Full Spine, Kinesiology, Gonstead

**KENNETH MINNICK, D.C.**
2606 S. Sheridan
Tulsa, OK 74129
(918) 835-4474
CHIROPRACTIC: F.SP., Diversified, Activator, Meric, Applied Kinesiology, Nutrition, Physical Therapy

**RICHARD LAWYER, D.C.**
715 W. Main #W
Jenks, OK 74037
(918) 299-1296
CHIROPRACTIC: Full Spine, Sacro Occipital Technique, Physical Therapy, Nutrition

**ALICE LONG, D.C.**
511 W. Third St.
Elk City, OK 73644
(405) 225-0155
CHIROPRACTIC: Orthopedics, Nutrition, Acupuncture, Activator, Applied Kinesiology, Colon Therapy, Physical Therapy, Hair Analysis, X-Rays

**MARTIN MEARS, D.C.**
2620 E. 2nd St.
Edmond, OK 73083
(405) 348-2226
CHIROPRACTIC: Sacro Occipital Technique, Cranial, Applied Kinesiology, Activator, Physical Therapy

## OREGON

**NORTH COAST CHIROPRACTIC CENTER**
679 E. Harbor Dr. #C
Warrenton, OR 97146
(503) 861-1661
CHIROPRACTIC: Sacro Occipital Technique, Thompson, Toftness, Diversified

**DAVID BRAMAN, D.C.**
18847 S.W. 84th
Tualatin, OR 97062
(503) 692-5260
CHIROPRACTIC: Applied Kinesiology, Full Spine, Nutrition, Activator, Physical Therapy

**LOYAL PARADIS, D.C.**
901 W. Centennial
Springfield, OR 97477
(503) 746-4122
CHIROPRACTIC: Palmer, Applied Kinesiology, Gonstead

**JEFFREY UTTER, D.C.**
3295 Triangle Dr. S. #160
Salem, OR 97302
(503) 364-0040
CHIROPRACTIC: Jennes, Toftness, COX, Sacro Occipital Technique, Laser Acupuncture

**ARN STRASSER, D.C.**
7904 S.E. 13th St.
Portland, OR 97202
(503) 231-1235
CHIROPRACTIC: Sacro Occipital Technique, Diversified, Holistic, MP, COX

**BETTER HEALTH CHIROPRACTIC CENTER**
RENA SANDLER, D.C.
1130 S.W. Morrison  Suite 301
Portland, OR 97214
(503) 222-2888
CHIROPRACTIC: Applied Kinesiology, Sacro Occipital Technique, Activator, Diversified, Extremities

**SANTO PULLELLA, D.C.**
748 S.E. 181st
Portland, OR 97233
(503) 232-4060
CHIROPRACTIC: Applied Kinesiology,
Sacro Occipital Technique, DNFT, Manner
Metabolic

**SALLY GREEN, D.C.**
2303 E. Burnside
Portland, OR 97214
(503) 239-7031
CHIROPRACTIC: Applied Kinesiology,
Cranial, Nutrition, Physical Therapy

**FRANK CALPENO, D.C.**
12223 N.E. Hoyt
Portland, OR 97230
(503) 255-3200
CHIROPRACTIC: Applied Kinesiology,
Sacro Occipital Technique, Homeopathy,
Cranial, Lab, Nutrition, DNFT, Acupuncture, Botanical

**MARK BURDELL, D.C.**
541 Park St.
Lebanon, OR 97355
(503) 451-1290
CHIROPRACTIC: Non Force, Applied
Kinesiology, Cranial, COX, Diversified

**LESLIE FEINBERG, D.C.**
633 E. Main St.
Hermiston, OR 97838
(503) 567-0200
CHIROPRACTIC: COX Chiromanis, Gonstead, Activator, Applied Kinesiology,
Sports Medicine, Physical Therapy, Myofacial

**SHARELL TRACY, D.C.**
59 Santa Clara
Eugene, OR 97404
(503) 689-0935
CHIROPRACTIC: Motion Palpation, Kinesiology, Pettibon, Thompson, Gonstead,
Palmer Toggle

**ARTHUR TICKNOR, D.C.**
1846 Pearl St.
Eugene, OR 97401
(503) 342-4216
CHIROPRACTIC: DNFT, Applied Kinesiology, Sacro Occipital Technique, Nutrition, Activator, Spinal Touch

**CHARLES SIMPSON, D.C.**
**RICHARD TILDEN, D.C.**
1250 Baseline
P.O. Box 507
Cornelius, OR 97113
(503) 357-3821
CHIROPRACTIC: Activator, Diversified,
Gonstead, Toftness, Sacro Occipital Technique

**THOMAS BOLERA, D.C.**
20330 S.E. Highway 212
Clackamas, OR 97015
(503) 658-5982
CHIROPRACTIC: Gonstead, Diversified,
Applied Kinesiology, Nutrition

**MARC HELLER, D.C.**
**JOHN KALB**
987 Siskiyou
Ashland, OR 97520
(503) 482-0625
CHIROPRACTIC: Applied Kinesiology,
Stressology, Toftness, Activator, Sacro
Occipital Technique, COX, Nutrition,
Electro Acupuncture

**HAZELFERN CHIROPRACTIC CLINIC**
BURT and RENEE ESPY, D.C.
7300 Hazelfern Rd.
Suite 201
Tigard, OR 97224
(503) 620-4174
CHIROPRACTIC: Nutritional Counseling
and Testing, Allergy Testing

**LAKE GROVE CHIROPRACTIC CLINIC**
DR. RENE O. ESPY
17125 S.W. Boones Ferry Rd.
Lake Oswego, OR 97034
(503) 636-0186
CHIROPRACTIC: Nutritional Counseling,
Acupressure, Applied Kinesiology

**PENNSYLVANIA**

**EVON BARVINCHACK, D.C.**
11142 Williamsport Pike
Greencastle, PA 17225
(717) 597-9470
CHIROPRACTIC: Sacro Occipital Technique, Orthopedics (FACO), TMJ, Sports
Injury

**GERALD H. SMITH, D.D.S.**
40 Court St.
Newtown, PA 18940
(215) 968-4781
DENTAL: TMJ, Orthodontics, Nutritional
Counseling, Craniopathy, Dental Orthopedics, Full Mouth Rehabilitation, Soft
Laser Acupuncture

**DONALD L. ROBBINS, D.M.D.**
340 North Pottstown Pike
Route 100
Exton, PA 19341
(215) 363-1980
DENTAL: TMJ

**DOUGLAS COLLINS, D.D.S.**
232 S. Burrowes St.
State College, PA 16801-4008
(814) 234-0921
DENTAL: TMJ, Oral Surgery

**RONALD W. NIKLAUS, D.D.S.**
3456 Trindle Rd.
CampHill, PA 17011
(717) 737-3353
DENTAL: TMJ Dysfunction, General
Dentistry, Oral Reconstruction

**JOSEPH OLIVETTI, D.D.S.**
Route 74 N.
Rd. 4
Dillsburg, PA 17019
(717) 432-3680
DENTAL: TMJ, General Dentistry

**GEORGE CHARLES, D.D.S.**
1151 Cornwall Rd.
Lebanon, PA 17042
(717) 273-4764
DENTAL: TMJ, General Dentistry, Head,
Neck and Shoulder Pain, Cranial Manipulation, Nutritional Counseling, Posture
Correction, Electric Acupuncture (Alpha
stim 2000)

**ANTHONY COOK, D.D.S.**
3007 Garrett Rd.
Drexel Hill, PA 19028
(215) 622-4400
DENTAL: TMJ, Orthodontics

**DALE C. RESUE, JR., D.M.D.**
21 N. Eagle Rd.
Havertown, PA 19083
(215) 789-0158
DENTAL: TMJ, General Dentistry

**JAMES BRADY, D.C.**
8010 Mill Creek Parkway
Levittown, PA 19054
(215) 945-8010
CHIROPRACTIC: Applied Kinesiology,
Sacro Occipital Technique, Activator,
Cranial Manipulation, Nutritional Coun-
seling, TMJ

**EDWARD BLUMENTHAL, D.C.**
444 North York Road
Hatboro, PA 19040
(215) 674-5599
CHIROPRACTIC: Pierce, X-Ray Motion
Spinal Analysis, Postural Correction,
Neuromuscular Structural Manipulation

**JOSEPH D. AVENT JR., D.D.S.**
7227 Hamilton Ave.
Pittsburg, PA 15208
(412) 243-3386
DENTAL: TMJ, General Dentistry

**DAVID BRUNO, D.C.**
1822 Mineral Spring Ave.
North Providence, PA 02904
(401) 353-5990
CHIROPRACTIC: Full Spine, Sacro Occipital Technique, Nutrition, Sports Medicine

**ALAN SCHWARTZ, D.C.**
4 Calvert St.
Newport, PA 02840
(401) 847-4224
CHIROPRACTIC: Applied Kinesiology,
COX, Activator, Full Body, Physical
Therapy, Nutrition

**WARREN FROBERG, D.C.**
Michael and River Roads
Yardley, PA 19067
(215) 295-4393
CHIROPRACTIC: Applied Kinesiology,
Sacro Occipital Technique, Cranial, Nutri-
tional Counseling

**WILLIAM LATTER, D.C.**
221 Old Eagle School Rd.
Wayne, PA 19087
(215) 293-1660
CHIROPRACTIC: NUCCA, COX, Disc
Traction, Activator, Applied Kinesiology

**THOMAS MISTRETTA, D.C.**
3362 E. State St.
Sharon, PA 16148
(412) 981-4550
CHIROPRACTIC: Grostic, COX, Gonstead,
Sacro Occipital Technique

**STEPHEN SHORE, D.C.**
5827 Ellsworth Ave.
Pittsburgh, PA 15232
(412) 363-2900
CHIROPRACTIC: HIO, Sacro Occipital
Technique, Diversified

**JOHN PIKULIN, D.C.**
221 Bridge St.
New Cumberland, PA 17070
(717) 774-5166
CHIROPRACTIC: Diversified, Sacro Occipital Technique, Applied Kinesiology,
Nutrition, Acupuncture

**ROBERT F. YANTIS, D.C.**
21 N. Fourth St.
McSherrystown, PA 17344
(717) 632-1012
CHIROPRACTIC: Spinal and Extremity
Manipulation, Applied Kinesiology, Nutrition

**THOMAS SNYDER, D.C.**
Rt. 209
P.O. Box 101
Brodheadsville, PA 18322
(717) 992-4787
CHIROPRACTIC: Full Spine, HIO, Ap-
plied Kinesiology, Orthopedics, Physical
Therapy

**199**

**CAROL DUNHAM, D.C.**
1715 W. Front St.
Berwick, PA 18603
(717) 759-2248
CHIROPRACTIC: Activator, Physical Therapy, Nutrition, Diversified, Sacro Occipital Technique

**BARRY R. GILLESPIE, D.C.**
193 Church Rd.
Devon, PA 19333
(215) 964-8967
DENTAL: Cranial Osteopathic Manipulation, Applied Kinesiology, TMJ

**YARDLEY CHIROPRACTIC CENTER**
DR. ARNO BURNIER, D.S.
DR. JOSEPH FASY
81 S. Main St.
Yardley, PA 19067
(215) 493-6589
CHIROPRACTIC: Education Programs, Motion Palpation

**INTERNATIONAL TREATMENT CENTER**
10 S. Leopard Rd.
Suite #1
Paoli, PA 19301
(215) 644-0136
PHYSICAL THERAPY: Electronic Acupuncture, Cold Laser Therapy, Biofeedback, Myofacial Release, Cranio-Sacral Therapy, TMJ

**ADVANCED CHIROPRACTIC CENTER**
326 Main St.
Red Hill, PA 18076
(215) 679-5915
CHIROPRACTIC: Applied Kinesiology, TMJ, Nutrition, Gonstead

**LUPOWITZ CHIROPRACTIC CENTER**
JEFFREY N. LUPOWITZ, D.C.
1217 W. Chester Pike
West Chester, PA 19380
(215) 692-6199
CHIROPRACTIC: Applied Kinesiology, Nutritional Counseling, Sacro Occipital Technique, Activator, Craniopathy, TMJ, Sports Injury

**DEEP MUSCLE THERAPY CENTER**
651 S. Gulph Rd.
King of Prussia, PA 19406
(215) 265-7939
DEEP MUSCLE THERAPY: Medical Examination, TMJ, Cranial Manipulation, Nutritional Consultation, Schooling in Corrective Muscle Therapy

**DR. STEPHEN DAVID SMITH**
Rte. 252 and Waynesborough Rd.
Paoli, PA 19301
(215) 647-2755
DENTAL: Homeopathy, Orthopedic Jaw Therapy, Physiotherapies, Jaw-Cranial Manipulation, Health-Centered Dentistry, Bruxism Control, Oral Metal-Current Screenings, Restorative and Cosmetic Dentistry

**DENNIS J. RED, D.M.D.**
6706 Carlisle Pike
Mechanicsburg, PA 17055
(717) 766-0600
DENTAL, PHYSICAL THERAPY: TMJ Orthopedics, Nutritional Counseling, Myofacial Release Techniques, Cranial Manipulation

**P. JAYALAKSHMI, M.D.**
6366 Sherwood Rd.
Philadelphia, PA 19151
(215) 473-4226
MEDICAL: Chelation-I.V., Allergy Control, Nutritional Counseling, Orthomolecular Psychiatry, Acupuncture, Colonics

**GARY S. COHEN, D.M.D.**
DEPARTMENT OF DENTAL MEDICINE
UNIVERSITY OF PENNSYLVANIA HOSPITAL
3400 Spruce St.
Philadelphia, PA 19104
(215) 662-3587
DENTAL: TMJ, Cranio-Facial Pain, Physical Therapy

**DONALD MANTELL, M.D.**
Rd. #1 Box 286
Evans City, PA 16033
(412) 776-5610
MEDICAL: Chelation Therapy, Clinical Ecology, Nutritional Counseling, Metabolic Programs for Degenerative Disease, Colonics, Massage Therapy

**ALAN D. HORWITZ, D.C.**
2555 Huntingdon Pike
Huntingdon Valley, PA 19006
(215) 947-0932
CHIROPRACTIC: Applied Kinesiology, Sacro Occipital Technique, Cranial Manipulation, Nutritional Counseling, Activator, Motion Palpation, TMJ

## RHODE ISLAND

**PAUL AARON, D.C.**
207 Waterman St.
Providence, RI 02906
(401) 272-1827
CHIROPRACTIC: Sacro Occipital Technique, Cranial Manipulation, TMJ, Nutritional Counseling

## SOUTH CAROLINA

**BRUCE H. KINNIE, D.D.S.**
7007 Brookfield Rd.
Columbia, SC 29206
(803) 788-8120
DENTAL: TMJ Dysfunction, Cranio-
acial Pain, Cervical Pain

**HERMAN PLEMMONS, D.C.**
425 Wade Hampton Blvd.
Greenville, SC 29609
(803) 271-1778
CHIROPRACTIC: Gonstead, Diversified,
Activator, Sacro Occipital Technique,
Meric, MP, Physical Therapy, Nutrition

**RICHARD BRANYON, D.C.**
419 College St.
P.O. Box 812
Greenville, SC 29601
(803) 232-6881
CHIROPRACTIC: Activator, Motion Palpation, Gonstead, Sacro Occipital Technique

**SUSAN BARKER, D.C.**
1568 Sunnyside Dr.
Columbia, SC 29204
(813) 738-0996
CHIROPRACTIC: Activator, Chiromanis,
Sacro Occipital Technique, Thompson,
Diversified

## TENNESSEE

**ROBERT T. KIRK, D.D.S.**
1154 Carter Drive
Chattanooga, TN 37415
(615) 870-4308
DENTAL: TMJ, Cranio-Facial Pain

**ARTHUR LENSGRAF, D.C.**
3827 Cleghorn Ave.
Nashville, TN 37215
(605) 383-5575
CHIROPRACTIC: HIO, Diversified, Applied
Kinesiology

**W.E. WENTWORTH, D.C.**
716 Highland
Jackson, TN 38301
(901) 427-5266
CHIROPRACTIC: Sacro Occipital Technique, Cranial, Harmonics, General Basic

**MELVIN MOONEY, D.C.**
6251 E. Brainerd Rd.
Chattanooga, TN 37421
(615) 894-1332
CHIROPRACTIC: Diversified, Kinesiology,
Activator, Physical Therapy

## TEXAS

**WELDON E. BELL, D.D.S.**
7022 Currin Drive
Dallas, TX 75230
(214) 368-5751
DENTAL: TMJ, Cranio-Facial Pain

**LORIN JACKOWSKI, D.C.**
22619 Aldine Westfield
Spring, TX 77373
(713) 350-0344
CHIROPRACTIC: Applied Kinesiology,
Sacro Occipital Technique, Activator,
Gonstead, Acupuncture, Nutrition

**A.R. MAULDIN, D.C.**
142 S. Lyndon B. Johnson Dr.
San Marcos, TX 78666
(512) 392-2876
CHIROPRACTIC: Applied Kinesiology,
Full Spine

**EUGENE GOLD, D.C.**
3405 W. Ave.
San Antonio, TX 78213
(512) 344-2880
CHIROPRACTIC: Activator, Sacro Occipital
Technique, Meridian Therapy, Nutrition,
Applied Kinesiology

**JAMES PAUL, D.C.**
2801 W. Parker Rd.
#4
Plano, TX 75023
(214) 596-3444
CHIROPRACTIC: Diversified, Applied
Kinesiology, NIMMO, Thompson, Gonstead,
Physical Therapy

**JOYCE M. PRUITT, D.C.**
5137-B 69th St.
Lubbock, TX 79424
(806) 794-6907
CHIROPRACTIC: Clinical Kinesiology

**SIDNEY ISDALE, D.C.**
**SCOTT ISDALE, D.C.**
2900 Trimmier
Killeen, TX 76541
(817) 699-4004
CHIROPRACTIC: Full Spine Diversified,
Activator, Applied Kinesiology, Physical
Therapy

**JAMES WELLINGTON, D.C.**
1308 Kingwood Drive
#140
Houston, TX 77339
(713) 358-1434
CHIROPRACTIC: Diversified, Activator,
Applied Kinesiology, Nutrition, F.SP.,
Physical Therapy

**MARYANN TOMKO, D.C.**
6910 Bellaire
#16
Houston, TX 77074
(713) 271-5105
CHIROPRACTIC: Applied   Kinesiology,
Sacro Occipital Technique, Logan, Activator,
Nutrition, COX

**BETH THOMPSON, D.C.**
6910 Bellaire Blvd.
#16
Houston, TX 77074
(713) 721-5105
CHIROPRACTIC: Applied   Kinesiology,
Activator, Gonstead, Nutrition, COX,
Physical Therapy

**NICK PROGULE, D.C.**
7645 Lon Point Rd.
Houston, TX 77055
(713) 683-8333
CHIROPRACTIC: Diversified, HIO, Activator, Applied Kinesiology, Nutrition,
Physical Therapy

**GUY LEUTWYLER, D.C.**
1212 Crosstimbers
Houston, TX 77022
(713) 697-1827
CHIROPRACTIC: Applied   Kinesiology,
Diversified, Activator, Nutrition

**HENRY JAEHNE, D.C.**
8602 Bellaire Blvd.
Houston, TX 77036
(713) 774-9595
CHIROPRACTIC: Full   Spine,   Applied
Kinesiology, Activator, Basic, Physiotherapy

**WINSTON GREENE, D.C.**
9724 Beechnut
101
Houston, TX 77036
(713) 995-1525
CHIROPRACTIC: Motion Palpation, Diversified F.SP.
Nutrition, Physical Therapy

**WINSTON GREENE, D.C.**
9724 Beechnut
#101
Houston, TX 77036
(713) 995-1525
CHIROPRACTIC: Motion Palpation, Diversified F.SP., Nutrition, Physical Therapy

**JOHN DEMARTINI, D.C.**
13155 Westheimer
#109-110
Houston, TX 77077
(713) 499-2424
CHIROPRACTIC: Applied   Kinesiology,
Diversified, Full Spine, Physical Therapy,
Nutrition

**RANDY BURDETT, D.C.**
10911 Chimney Rock
Houston, TX 77096
(713) 723-1204
CHIROPRACTIC: Diversified,   Physical
Therapy, Nutrition, COX, Cranial, Applied
Kinesiology

**DON RICE, D.C.**
6801 McCart
Fort Worth, TX 76133
(817) 481-7025
CHIROPRACTIC: Activator,   Applied
Kinesiology, Diversified, Nutrition

**JAMES BUCKNER, D.C.**
1313 Crestlane Dr.
Duncanville, TX 75137
(214) 296-1879
CHIROPRACTIC: Full Spine, Activator,
Applied Kinesiology, Sacro Occipital Technique, Physical Therapy

**JOLYN ENGLISH, D.C.**
501 W. Hondo St.
Devine, TX 78016
(512) 663-4453
CHIROPRACTIC: Sacro Occipital Tech-
nique, TMJ, Applied Kinesiology, CK,
Activator, Nutrition, Gonstead, Physical
Therapy

**ACCENT HEALTH CARE CENTER**
TY TYCOTT, D.C.
9115 Forest Lane
Dallas, TX 75243
(214) 231-9391
CHIROPRACTIC: Diversified, Activator,
Applied Kinesiology, Physical Therapy,
Extensilizer Treatment

**DAVID CLEMENTS, D.C.**
5555 Preston Oaks #3
Dallas, TX 75240
(214) 788-4555
CHIROPRACTIC: Applied   Kinesiology,
Activator, Nutrition, NIMMO, Livecell
Analysis

**C.W. FAW, D.C.**
RUBY PERKINS FAW
10926 Leopard #C
Corpus Christi, TX 78410
(512) 241-5744
CHIROPRACTIC: Meric, Gonstead, Sacro
Occipital Technique, Full Spine, Physical
Therapy

**MIKE VANDEWALE, D.C.**
3624 N. Hills Dr.
A-101
Austin, TX 78731
(512) 343-0700
CHIROPRACTIC: Gonstead,   Palmer,
Sacro Occipital Technique, Diversified

MARK SANDERS, D.C.
STEPHEN SUMMERS, D.C.
PATRICK CASEY
4804 Grover Ave.
Austin, TX 78756
(512) 458-5378
CHIROPRACTIC: Applied Kinesiology,
Sacro Occipital Technique, Activator, MP,
Diversified, Body Work, Chiropractic
Lectures, Wellness Class

ARTHUR PETERSON, D.C.
CONNIE PETERSON, D.C.
HART PETERSON, D.C.
2105 Justin Lane #116
Austin, TX 78757
(512) 454-3533
CHIROPRACTIC: Applied Kinesiology,
Full Spine, COX, Sacro Occipital Technique,
Cranial, Physical Therapy, Nutrition

STEVEN KLAYMAN, D.C.
950 Westlake High Dr.
Austin, TX 78746
(512) 327-9777
CHIROPRACTIC: Applied Kinesiology,
Sacro Occipital Technique, Diversified,
Acupuncture, Physical Therapy, COX,
Gonstead, NIMMO

FRANK PETERS, D.C.
4020 W. 50th
Amarillo, TX 79109
(806) 352-2721
CHIROPRACTIC: Applied Kinesiology,
Sacro Occipital Technique, Activator,
Diversified, Gonstead

CHRONIC PAIN ASSOCIATES, P.C.
DR. JOSEPH A. KLEINKORT, D.C.
4499 Medical Drive
Suite 380
San Antonio, TX 78229
(512) 692-0786
PHYSICAL THERAPY: TMJ, Manipula-
tion, Soft Laser Acupuncture, TENS,
Electro Medicine, Sacro Occipital Technique,
Acuscope, Alphastim

D.J. FONG, D.D.S
6214 S.W. 34th
Amarillo, TX 79109
(806) 355-4421
DENTAL: Nutrition, Cranio-Sacral Treatment, SOT, Applied Kinesiology

## UTAH

ELDON ST. JEOR, D.D.S
2063 E. 3900 S.
Salt Lake City, UT 84124
(801) 278-2855
DENTAL: TMJ, General Dentistry

JAMES VAN SLOOTENN, D.C.
3428 S. 2300 E.
Salt Lake City, UT 84109
(801) 486-9201
CHIROPRACTIC: Logan Basic, Motion
Palpation, Applied Kinesiology

CHARLES CHAMBERS, D.C.
837 E. 2100 S.
Salt Lake City, UT 84105
(801) 484-2596
CHIROPRACTIC: Full Spine, Gonstead,
Applied Kinesiology, Activator

RODNEY DAVIS, D.C.
5255 S. State St.
Murray, UT 84107
(801) 268-9131
CHIROPRACTIC: Full Spine Palmer
Diversified, Gonstead, Applied Kinesiology, Physical Therapy

## VERMONT

ROBERT J. MILLER, D.D.S.
129 Elm St.
Bennington, VT 05201
(802) 442-9500
DENTAL: TMJ

HARRIS SNOPARSKY, D.C.
4 San Remo Dr.
South Burlington, VT 05401
(802) 658-6092
CHIROPRACTIC: Sacro Occipital Technique, Activator, NIMMO, Diversified,
Nutrition

MAURICE CYR, D.C.
245 Stratton Rd.
Rutland, VT 05701
(802) 775-6961
CHIROPRACTIC: MPI, Gonstead, Thompson, Activator, Nutrition, Physical Therapy,
Applied Kinesiology

## VIRGINIA

DR. RICHARD D. FISCHER
4222 Evergreen Lane
Annandale, VA 22003
(703) 256-4441
DENTAL: TMJ, Dental Cranial Treatment,
Dental Homeopathy, Nutritional Counseling, Applied Kinesiology, Auriculotherapy

WILLIAM J. MCGARRY, D.D.S.
307-F Maple Ave. W.
Vienna, VA 22180
(804) 281-1090
DENTAL: TMJ

**PHILIP H. MYONG, D.D.S.**
5217 Grantham St.
Springfield, VA 22151
(804) 978-7770
DENTAL: TMJ

**CHARLES MASARSKY, D.C.**
**DARION WEBER, D.C.**
301 Maple Ave.
Sect. 3, #H
Vienna, VA 22180
(703) 938-6441
CHIROPRACTIC: Diversified, Applied
Kinesiology, Motion Palpation, Nutrition

**GURUTRANG SINGH KHALSA, D.C.**
11890-A Sunrise Valley Dr.
Reston, VA 22091
(703) 476-1020
CHIROPRACTIC: Applied Kinesiology,
Nutrition, Diversified

**DENNIS SIEVERS, D.C.**
7865 Heritage Dr.
Annandale, VA 22003
(703) 642-5717
CHIROPRACTIC: Applied Kinesiology,
BEST, Sacro Occipital Technique, PST,
COX, Gonstead, RT, Activator, Physical
Therapy

**BONNIE SHAPIRO, D.C.**
5101-A Backlick Rd.
Annandale, VA 22003
(703) 642-8527
CHIROPRACTIC: Àctivator, Applied Kinesiology, NIMMO, Nutrition, Thompson

**MOWLES CHIROPRACTIC CLINIC**
RICHARD A. MOWLES, D.C., D.I.C.A.K.
4326 Brambleton Ave., S.W.
Roanoke, VA 24018
(703) 989-4584
CHIROPRACTIC: Nutritional Counseling,
Applied Kinesiology

**WASHINGTON**

**DR. RUSS BORNEMAN**
Burton Bldg., Suite 211
Anacortes, WA 98221
(206) 293-8451
DENTAL: TMJ, Dental Orthopedics, Orthodontics, Mercury Free Dentistry, Children's Dentistry

**SEATTLE HEALTH CLINIC**
DR. LOUISA L. WILLIAMS
425 Broadway (Broadway Market)
Seattle, WA 98102
(206) 322-9355
CHIROPRACTIC: Sacro Occipital Tech-
nique, Applied Kinesiology, TMJ, Cranial
Manipulation, Psychotherapy, Colonics,
Massage, Nutritional Counseling

**GERALD OXFORD, D.C.**
116 W. Third St.
Wapato, WA 98951
(509) 877-4114
CHIROPRACTIC: Palmer, Gonstead,
Applied Kinesiology, Sacro Occipital Technique, Activator, TMJ, Cranio Manipulation, Consultant: Dept. of Labor & Industry

**JACK ELIVIDGE, D.C.**
E. 15803 Sprague
Veradale, WA 99037
(509) 928-0474
CHIROPRACTIC: Activator, Applied
Kinesiology, Motion Palpation, Palmer
Pkg.

**KENNETH DAY, D.C.**
9328 271st St. N.W.
Stanwood, WA 98292
(206) 629-2650
CHIROPRACTIC: Sacro Occipital Technique, Palmer, Stillwagon, Thompson,
Diversified

**DAVID SCHEER, D.C.**
17234 Pacific Highway
Seattle, WA 98188
(206) 246-8830
CHIROPRACTIC: Applied Kinesiology,
Sacro Occipital Technique, Diversified,
NIMMO

**GARY BRETOW, D.C.**
2004 Fairview Ave.
Seattle, WA 98121
(206) 623-6800
CHIROPRACTIC: Pettibon, Gonstead,
Thompson, Diversified, Sacro Occipital
Technique

**LAKE UNION CHIROPRACTIC CLINIC**
CHRISTINE A. MESHEW
4464 Stone Way North
Seattle, WA 98103
(206) 632-9600
CHIROPRACTIC: Sacro Occipital Technique, Applied Kinesiology, Cranial Manipulation, TMJ, Nutritional Counseling,
Allopathic, NLP Counseling

**BERNARD JANKELSON, D.M.D.**
720 Olive Way
Suite 800
Seattle, WA 98101
(206) 622-2121
DENTAL: TMJ, Cranio-facial Pain

**JAMES GOULD, D.C.**
709 S. Lilly Rd.
Olympia, WA 98501
(206) 456-4488
CHIROPRACTIC: Kinesiology, Diversified,
COX, Activator, Logan

## PUYALLUP CHIROPRACTIC CLINIC
1203 E. Main St.
Puyllup, WA 98371
(206) 845-0543
CHIROPRACTIC: Full Spine, Palmer, Gonstead, Applied Kinesiology, Thompson, Stressology, Activator, Motion Palpation, Diversified

## FREDERICK BOMONTI, D.C.
12511 S. Meridian
Puyallup, WA 98373
(206) 848-1584
CHIROPRACTIC: Diversified, Sacro Occipital Technique, Activator

## ELEANOR DUBEY, D.C.
1702 E. 4th Ave.
Olympia, WA 98506
(206) 943-4333
CHIROPRACTIC: Diversified Full Spine, Sports Injury, Nutrition, Sacro Occipital Technique, Toftness, Colon Therapy

## EDWARD SULLIVAN, D.C.
307 E. Division St.
Mount Vernon, WA 98271
(206) 336-9512
CHIROPRACTIC: Gonstead, Palmer, COX, Sacro Occipital Technique, Thompson

## KRIS DEXTER, D.C.
900 E. Nelson Rd.
Moses Lake, WA 98837
(509) 765-0239
CHIROPRACTIC: Toftness, Chiromanis, Sacro Occipital Technique

## CARSON ODEGARD, D.C.
822 S. Sixth St.
Kirkland, WA 98033
(206) 827-4646
CHIROPRACTIC: Gonstead, Motion Palpation, Kinesiology

## RICHARD BAKER, D.C.
10830 Kent-Kangley Rd.
Kent, WA 98031
(206) 854-3040
CHIROPRACTIC: Activator, Sacro Occipital Technique, Cranial, Pettibon, COX, Thompson

## DOYLE and GITHENS, D.C.
16923 96th Ave. N.E.
Bothell, WA 98011
(206) 485-7507
CHIROPRACTIC: Toftness, Activator, Applied Kinesiology, Gonstead, COX

## SURESH RANCHOD, D.C.
14862 Lake Hills Blvd.
Bellevue, WA 98007
(206) 747-5622
CHIROPRACTIC: Sacro Occipital Technique, COX, Applied Kinesiology, Diversified, Toftness

## CARL JELSTRUP, D.C.
10230 N.E. Tenth Ave.
Bellevue, WA 98004
(206) 455-5390
CHIROPRACTIC: Sacro Occipital Technique, Cranial, Toftness, TMJ Dental, Applied Kinesiology

## STOUT CHIROPRACTIC CARE CENTER
ELAINE C. STOUT-TIDWELL, D.C.
432 West Ave.
Arlington, WA 98223
(206) 435-9455
CHIROPRACTIC: TMJ, Craniopathy, Organic Dysfunction, Chiropractic Manipulation Reflex Technique, Extremity, Orthdontics, Nutritional Counseling and Testing

## JAY GOODWIN, D.C.
16827 35th Ave. N.E.
Arlington, WA 98223
(206) 653-4626
CHIROPRACTIC: Toftness, Sacro Occipital Technique, Activator

## MICHAEL BRENEMAN, D.C.
3210 Smokey Point Blvd.
Arlington, WA 98223
(206) 652-0211
CHIROPRACTIC: Applied Kinesiology, Activator, Thompson, Gonstead

## JAMES E. CARLSON, D.D.S.
13401 Bell Red Rd.
Bellevue, WA 98005
(206) 746-0021
DENTAL: TMJ, Cranio-Facial Pain, Reconstructive Dentistry

## MERLE LOUDEN, D.D.S.
530 Valley Mall Pkwy
East Wenatchee, WA 98802
(509) 884-7151
DENTAL: TMJ, Dental Orthopedics, Orthodontics

## WILLIAM J. PLOGER, D.D.S.
1207 N. 145th St.
Seattle, WA 98133
(206) 364-0720
DENTAL: Dental Stress and Tension, Orthopedic, Orthodontic, Nutritional Guidance

**ARMAND V DE FELICE, D.D.S.**
N. 4703 Maple
Spokane, WA 99208
(509) 327-7719
DENTAL: TMJ, Cranio-Facial Pain, General Dentistry, Mercury Free Fillings

**FALL CITY CHIROPRACTIC CENTER**
River St.
P.O. Box 189
Fall City, WA 98024

**FALL CITY CHIROPRACTIC CENTER**
River St.
P.O. Box 189
Fall City, WA 98024
(206) 222-5125
CHIROPRACTIC: Sacro Occipital Technique, Applied Kinesiology

**JOHN O. STOUTENBURG, D.C.**
17320 135th Ave. N.E.
Suite D
Woodinville, WA 98072
(206) 483-5454
CHIROPRACTIC: Applied Kinesiology, Nutritional Counseling

**RUNAR D. JOHNSON, D.D.S.**
321 N. Sequim Ave.
Sequim, WA 98382
(206) 683-4850
DENTAL: TMJ, Cranio-Facial Pain, General Dentistry, Mercury Free Fillings, Nutritional Counseling, Cranial Manipulation

**LAVAR RINIKER, D.D.S.**
121 3rd Ave.
Suite 220
Kirkland, WA 98033-6151
(206) 822-6003
DENTAL: TMJ, Cranio-Facial Pain, Dental Orthopedics, Full Mouth Restoration, Myo-monitor, Kinesiograph, Mercury Free Fillings

### WEST VIRGINIA

**JOHN H. GERATH, D.C.**
Rt. 1 Box 217A
Jane Lew, WV 26378
(304) 884-7189
CHIROPRACTIC: Sacro Occipital Technique, Cranial Manipulation

### WISCONSIN

**HEALTH CENTERED CARE**
JOHN D. LAUGHLIN, III, D.D.S.
375 Kinnie St. Box 900
Ellsworth, WI 54011
(715) 273-3503
DENTAL: TMJ, Dental Orthopedics, Orthodontics, General Dentistry, Preventive Therapy, Dental Cranial Therapy

**FRED KRIEMELMEYER, D.D.S.**
3143 State Rd.
Lacrosse, WI 54601
(608) 788-0306
DENTAL: Dental Craniopathy, Orthopedics, Orthodontics, TMJ, Nutritional Counseling, Dental Myotherapy

**DANIEL WITKOWSKI, D.D.S**
100 W. Monroe St.
Port Washington, WI 53074
(414) 284-7151
DENTAL: TMJ

**MICHAEL A. HANSEN, D.C.**
1400 S. Green Bay Rd.
Suite 102
Racine, WI 53406
(414) 639-7223
CHIROPRACTIC: Sacro Occipital Technique

**DAVID STOIBER, D.C.**
211 W. Grand Ave.
Wisconsin Rapids, WI 54494
(715) 424-4646
CHIROPRACTIC: COX, Pettibon, Activator, Sacro Occipital Technique, Diversified

**NELSON CHIROPRACTIC CENTER**
DR. MELISSA V. NELSON, D.C.
30 N. 18th Ave.
Sturgeon Bay, WI 54235
(414) 743-7153
CHIROPRACTIC: Applied Kinesiology, Clinical Nutrition, Rolfing, Activator, Massage Therapy, Family Counseling

**J.G. MOELLENDORF, D.C.**
1140 Egg Harbor Rd.
Sturgeon Bay, WI 54235
(414) 743-2126
CHIROPRACTIC: Applied Kinesiology, COX, Sacro Occipital Technique, CMRT

**PAUL and BRAD SMITH, D.C.**
1001 S. Whitney Way
Madison, WI 53711
(608) 274-6200
CHIROPRACTIC: Gonstead, Sacro Occipital Technique, Cranial, Basic, Nutrition

**HANS JEROSCH, D.C.**
2430 E. Washington Ave.
Madison, WI 53704
(608) 244-1740
CHIROPRACTIC: Toftness, Gonstead, Applied Kinesiology, Sacro Occipital Technique, F.SP. Specific

**KEN and URBAN STURGIS, D.C.**
1624 E. Mason St.
Green Bay, WI 54302
(414) 465-0400
CHIROPRACTIC: Gonstead, MPI, Diversified, Sacro Occipital Technique, NIMMO, Full Spine

**J & R CHIROPRACTIC OFFICE, D.C.**
1075 Brookwood Dr.
Green Bay, WI 54304
(414) 494-6601
CHIROPRACTIC: Gonstead, Activator, Applied Kinesiology, COX

**MARTIN HAZUKA, D.C.**
1768 Main St.
Greenbay, WI 54302
(414) 468-4755
CHIROPRACTIC: Sacro Occipital Technique, Basic, Applied Kinesiology

**STEVEN J. CARINI, D.D.S.**
222 Franklin St.
Port Washington, WI 53074
(414) 284-2662
DENTAL: TMJ, Cranio-Facial Pain, General Dentistry

**JENSEN CHIROPRACTIC CENTER**
JAN M. JENSEN, D.C.
4701 W. National
Milwaukee, WI 53214
(414) 645-1616
CHIROPRACTIC: Applied Kinesiology, Macrobiotic Counseling and Nutritional Evaluation, Acupressure, TMJ, Cranial Manipulation

## CANADA

**WHOLE HEALTH CENTER**
DR. CAROLYN A. ZIMMERMAN
10203-121 St.
Edmonton, Alberta
Canada T5N 1K6
(403) 482-7175
CHIROPRACTIC: Sacro Occipital Technique, Cranial Manipulation, Nutritional Counseling, Hair Analysis, Acupressure, Life Style Management

**CHAMBUL CHIROPRACTIC GROUP**
BORYS M. CHAMBUL, D.C.
9 Bloor St. E.
Toronto, Ontario
Canada M4W 1A3
(416) 961-6660
CHIROPRACTIC: Applied Kinesiology, Cold Laser Therapy, Meridian Therapy, Myopulse, Cranial Manipulation, Nutritional Counseling, Life Style Management

**MONICA L. TRACY, D.C.**
501 - 207 W. Hastings St.
Vancouver, B.C.
Canada V6B 1H7
(604) 688-1625
CHIROPRACTIC: Sacro Occipital Technique and Associated Techniques

**DONALD G. MARSHALL, D.D.S.**
4347 W. 10th Ave.
Vancouver, BC V6N 2K6
(604) 228-9041
DENTAL: General Dentistry, Stress Management and Life Style Management, Nutritional Counseling

**DR. WOLFGANG P. KLIEM**
6154 Fraser St.
Vancouver, BC V5W 3A1
(604) 321-6704
CHIROPRACTIC: Sacro Occipital Technique, TMJ, Cranial Manipulation, Applied Kinesiology, Motion Palpation, Sports Injury, Zindler Technique, Extremities

**DR. RAINER ZINDLER**
6154 Fraser St.
Vancouver, BC V5W 3A1
(604) 321-6704
CHIROPRACTIC: Sacro Occipital Technique, TMJ, Sports Injuries, Cranial Manipulation, Zindler Technique, Extremities

**BRIAN STRUKOFF, D.D.S.**
202-45625 Hodgins Ave.
Chilliwack, B.C
Canada V2P 1P2
(604) 792-9371
DENTAL: TMJ, Dental Orthopedics, Orthodontics

**GORDON L. McMURRAY, D.D.S.**
Box 490
125 First St.
Parksville, B.C. Y0R 2S0
(604) 248-6232
DENTAL: Orthodontics, Cranifacial, Neck and TMJ Pain

**BRIGITTE FAAS, D.C.**
1986 Queen St.
Suite 207
Toronto, Ontario
Canada M4L 1H9
(416) 698-7070
CHIROPRACTIC: Sacro Occipital Technique, Cranial Manipulation, TMJ

**HELEN M. PEEL, D.C.**
108 Water St.
Port Perry, Ontario
Canada L0B 1N0
(416) 985-3702
CHIROPRACTIC: Sacro Occipital Technique, Cranial Manipulation, TMJ

**REVA BATHIE, D.C.**
108 Water St.
Port Perry, Ontario
Canada L0B 1N0
(416) 985-3702
CHIROPRACTIC: Sacro Occipital Technique, Cranial Manipulation, TMJ

**L.R. MOORHEAD, D.C.**
738 Kildonan Drive
Winnipeg, Manitoba
Canada R2K 2E3
(204) 222-2969
CHIROPRACTIC: Sacro Occipital Technique, Cranial Manipulation

**W.B. CHAMPION, D.C.**
510 10th St.
Wainwright, Alberta
Canada T0B 4P0
(403) 842-3301
CHIROPRACTIC: Sacro Occipital Technique

**DOUGLAS R. HALL, D.C.**
P.O. Box 124
Peace River, Alberta
Canada T0H 2X0
(403) 624-2121
CHIROPRACTIC: Sacro Occipital Technique

**D. GORDON HASICK, D.C.**
5005 Elbow Drive, S.W.
Suite 201
Calgary, Alberta
Canada T2S 2T6
(403) 243-0155
CHIROPRACTIC: Sacro Occipital Technique

## AUSTRALIA

## NEW SOUTH WALES

**KEITH BASTIAN, D.C.**
P.O. Box 333
Forster, N.S.W., Aus. 2428
(06) 554-7388
CHIROPRACTIC: SOT

**SCOTT PARKER, D.C.**
83 Walker Street
Casino, N.S.W., Aus.
(066) 62-4077
CHIROPRACTIC: SOT

**KENNETH R. COOPER, D.C.**
21 Delany Ave.
Narrabri, N.S.W., Aus. 2390
(06) 792-2022
CHIROPRACTIC: SOT

**PETER COWIE, D.C.**
P.O. BOX 428
Pennant Hills, N.S.W., Aus. 2120
84-7090
CHIROPRACTIC: SOT

**JEFFERSON G. TAYLOR, D.C.**
206 Blaxland Road
Ryde, N.S.W., Aus. 2112
808-1122
CHIROPRACTIC: SOT

**VANESSA-ANNE TEO, D.C.**
3 River Terrace
Tweed Heads, N.S.W., Aus. 2485
(075) 36 5852
CHIROPRACTIC: SOT

**JOHN CARP, D.C.**
Greendale Road
Wallacia, N.S.W., Aus. 2750
CHIROPRACTIC: SOT

**JOHN PETTIT, D.C.**
201 Great Western Hiway
Wentworth Falls, N.S.W., Aus. 2782
(04) 757-3187
CHIROPRACTIC: SOT

**ARTHUR CIMIJOTTA, D.C.**
18 Karani Ave.
West Guilford, N.S.W., Aus. 2161
(02) 632-8091
CHIROPRACTIC: SOT

## QUEENSLAND

**L.J. CLARK, D.C.**
23 Bowen Street
Capalaba, Brisbain, Aus. 4157
CHIROPRACTIC: SOT

**DOUGLAS B. HART, D.C.**
860 Old Cleveland Road
Carina, Aus. 4152
(07) 398-3876
CHIROPRACTIC: SOT

**BRUCE E. MACDONALD, D.C.**
14 Stewart Street
Kilcoy, Aus. 4515
(07) 197-1747
CHIROPRACTIC: SOT

**TERRELL G. KLEMA, D.C.**
27 Webb Street
kippa-ring, Aus. 4019
(07) 284-0866
CHIROPRACTIC: SOT

**ALLAN L. LAMBERT, D.C.**
76 Currie Street
Nambour, Aus. 4560
(07) 141-3611
CHIROPRACTIC: SOT

**LINDA B. POWER, D.C.**
76 Currie Street
Nambour, Aus. 4560
(07) 141-3611
CHIROPRACTIC:   SOT

**KENNETH W. BARNES, D.C.**
17 Hubert
South Townsville, Aus. 4810
(07) 772-2895
CHIROPRACTIC:   SOT

**RONALD W. HASLETT, D.C.**
497 Gynipie Road
Strathpine, Aus.
CHIROPRACTIC:   SOT

**B. A. ROCK. D.C.**
31 Healy Street
Toowoomba, Aus. 4350
(07) 635-7291
CHIROPRACTIC:   SOT

**G. I. PAPWORTH, D.C.**
26 Alfred Street
Woody Point, Aus. 4019
(07) 284-1090
CHIROPRACTIC:   SOT

### SOUTH AUSTRALIA

**RONDA V.B. WALLIS, D.C.**
39 Russel Road
Adelaide, Aus. 5076
(08) 336-5553
CHIROPRACTIC:   SOT

**G. WORTHINGTON-EYRE, D.C.**
80 Beach Road
Christies Beach, Aus. 5165
(08) 384-3919
CHIROPRACTIC:   SOT

**KYM A. WILLIAMS, D.C.**
421 Payneham Road
Felixtowe, Aus. 5070
(08) 336-6461
CHIROPRACTIC:   SOT

**WILLIAN A. WILLIAMS, D.C.**
421 Payneham Road
Felixtowe, Aus. 5070
(08) 336-6461
CHIROPRACTIC:   SOT

**WILLIAM D. LOGAN, D.C.**
315 Glen Osmond Road
Glenunga, Aus. 5064
(08) 79-7318
19 George Street
Moonta, Aus. 5558
(088) 25-2822
CHIROPRACTIC:   SOT

**DIANNE BAILEY, D.C.**
Room 1, 94 King Road
Hyde Park, Aus. 5061
(08) 272-5322
CHIROPRACTIC:   SOT

**NEVILLE CREED, D.C.**
56 Bay Road
Mount Gambier, Aus. 5290
(087) 25-3755
CHIROPRACTIC:   SOT

**LINDA R. TURLEY, D.C.**
P.O. Box 825
Mt. Gambier, Aus. 5290
(087) 25-3755
CHIROPRACTIC:   SOT

**D. DICKMANN, D.C.**
35 Launer Ave.
Rostrevor, Aus. 5073
(08) 337-8572
CHIROPRACTOR:   SOT

**STEVEN M. VOZZO, D.C.**
205 Henley Beach Road
Torrensville, Aus. 5031
CHIROPRACTIC:   SOT

### VICTORIA

**LARRAINE STEWART, D.C**
204 Mill Street
Ballarat, Aus. 3350
(053) 32-6526
CHIROPRACTIC:   SOT

**D LOVETT, D.C.**
27 View Street
Bendigo, Aus. 3550
(054) 43-9744
CHIROPRACTIC:   SOT

**LISA LOVETT, D.C.**
4 McLaren Street
Bendigo, Aus. 3550
(054) 43-3544
CHIROPRACTIC:   SOT

**A. MARK POSTLES, D.C.**
21 View Street
Bendigo, Aus. 3550
(054) 43-9744
CHIROPRACTIC:   SOT

**L. V. STASINOWSKY, D.C.**
30 Well Street
Brighton, Aus. 3186
(03) 592-7695
CHIROPRACTIC:   SOT

**F.R. JEFFERY, D.C.**
45 Princes Highway
Dandenong, Aus. 3175
792-4201
CHIROPRACTIC:   SOT

**MICHAEL DUNN, D.C.**
1046 Doncaster Road
Doncaster East, Aus. 3109
842-1731
CHIROPRACTOR: SOT

**KENNETH J. LEYONHJELM, D.C.**
63 Nish Street
Echuca, Aus. 3625
(054) 82-1477
CHIROPRACTOR: SOT

**GAVIN R. JAMES, D.C.**
300 Albert Road
South Melbourne, Aus. 3205
(03) 690-2582
CHIROPRACTOR: SOT

**LOUIS ROTMAN, D.C.**
73 Kensington Road
South Yarra, Aus. 3141
(03) 241-8002
CHIROPRACTOR: SOT

**CHRISTOPHER G. MURRAY, D.D.S.**
20 Collins Street Coats Bldg.
4th Floor
Melbourne, Aus. 3000
DENTAL: TMJ, Head, Neck, and facial
pain, Reconstruction

**ROBERT D. WENBAN, D.C.**
417 Hampton Street
Melbourne, Aus.
CHIROPRACTOR: SOT

**KIM BAUGHURST, D.C.**
9 Haigh Street
Moe, Aus. 3825
(051) 27 5757
CHIROPRACTIC: SOT

**ANTHONY R. HART, D.C.**
Marine Road
San Remo, Aus. 3825
(05) 678-5459
CHIROPRACTOR: SOT

**WILLIAM MACPHERSON, D.C.**
55-57 Argyle Street
Traralgon, Aus. 3844
(05) 174-1891
CHIROPRACTOR: SOT

**TREVOR D. CREED, D.C.**
1 Banyan Street
Warrnambool, Aus. 3280
(05) 562-1877
CHIROPRACTOR: SOT

**JOANNE P. JENNINGS, D.C.**
3 Banyan Street
Warrnambool, Aus. 3280
(05) 562-1877
CHIROPRACTOR: SOT

**W. R. JENNINGS, D.C.**
1-3 Banyan Street
Warrnambool, Aus. 3280
(05) 562-1877
CHIROPRACTIC: SOT

**ERIC O. DOWKER, D.C.**
296 Grimshaw Street
Watsonia, Aus. 3087
(03) 434-3086
CHIROPRACTIC: SOT

**A. J. H. POWELL, D.C.**
296 Grimshaw Street
Watsonia, Aus. 3087
(03) 434-3086
CHIROPRACTIC: SOT

## DENMARK

**KIROPRAKTISK KLINIK
JOSEPH SHAFER, D.C.**
Lyngby Hovedgade 60
Lyngby, Denmark 2800
02 87 99 00
CHIROPRACTIC: Applied Kinesiology,
Craniopathy, TMJ, Nutritional Counseling

## ENGLAND

**JONATHAN M. HOWAT, D.C.**
14 Holyoake Road
Headington, Oxford 0X3 8AE
Oxford 61802
CHIROPRACTIC: SOT, TMJ, Cranial
Manipulation

**GILBERT M. MEAL, D.C.**
5, Stour Road
Christchurch Dorset, BH231PL England
44 02 02 48 32 81
CHIROPRACTIC: Applied Kinesiology,
Sports Injuries, Allergies, Nutritional
Counseling, Ergonomics

**RICHARD LAWSON, D.C.**
82, Lowlands Road
Harrow HAL 3AN England
CHIROPRACTIC:

**RICHARD L. COOK, D.C.**
82, Lowlands Road
Harrow, Middx., HA1 3AN, England
01 86 46 76 8
CHIROPRACTIC: Applied Kinesiology,
Craniopathy, TMJ, Pediatrics, Chiropractic
Pain Control

**210**

**WEST**
Dr. E.C. Hamlyn, M.B., CLB
Dorothy West
Rutt House
Ivybridge, Devon PL210DQ
England
0752-892792
MEDICAL: Homeopathy, Clinical Ecology,
Orthomolecular Medicine, Food and Che-
mical Allergies, Applied Kinesiology,
Intradermal Titration Testing

## FRANCE

**PHILIPPE DU PONT, D.C.**
Place De La Marie
Argeles-Gazost, 65400, France
CHIROPRACTIC: SOT

**CHANTAL REDON, D.C.**
4 Blvd. Foch
Grenoble, 38100, France
76 46 96 83
CHIROPRACTIC: SOT

**ALAIN GEHIN, D.C.**
3 Rue Coislin
Metz, 57000, France
87 14 07 95
CHIROPRACTIC: SOT, Cranial Manipulation Head, Neck and Facial Pain
**HENRIETTA FREY, D.C.**
28 Rue De L'ancien Courrier
Montpellier, 34000, France
67 60 54 69
CHIROPRACTIC: SOT

**MICHEL PLANTIER, D.C.**
2 Rue De Leningrad
Paris, 8, France
45 22 75 07
CHIROPRACTIC: SOT

**LOUIS NAHMANI, D.D.S.**
236 Saint Germain Blvd.
Paris, 75007, France
(33) 548-1300
DENTAL: TMJ, General Dentistry, Cranio-Facial Pain

**JEAN-PIERRE BOURSETTE, D.C.**
43 Avenue Marino
Sigolene, 43600, France
71 66 63 47
CHIROPRACTIC: SOT

**CHANTAL JOLLIOT, D.C.**
22, Av Du General De Gaulle
Strasbourg, 67000, France
88 61 68 82
CHIROPRACTIC: SOT, Cranial Manipulation

**MICHELINE ROUGEBEC, D.C.**
17 Bis Rue Georget
Tours, 37000, France
47 37 88 02
CHIROPRACTIC: SOT

**RICHARD C. MELDENER, D.C.**
49 Rue Des Mathurines
Paris, 75008, France
12 65 87 20
CHIROPRACTIC: Applied Kinesiology,
Sacro Occipital Technic

## INDIA

**DRS. MANU and HELENE SHAH**
P.O. Box 339
Margao, Goa 403 601
OSTEOPATHIC: Cranial Manipulation,
Nutritional Counseling, SOT, TMJ, Acu-
puncture, Educational Programs on Natu-
ral Healing, Treatment of Degenerative
Diseases, Total Holistic International
Health Center

## PHILIPPINES

**JAMESON T. UY, D.C.**
6 Molave Street
Forbes Park, Makati M.M., Philippines
817-0601
CHIROPRACTIC: Sacro Occipital Technic, Acupuncture, Applied Kinesiology

## SCOTLAND

**DR. JAN DE VRIES**
Auchenkyle Southwoods
Troon, Scotland
02 92 31 14 14
MEDICAL: Sacro Occipital Technic, Al-
ternative Care, Orthomolecular Psychiatry,
Applied Kinesiology, Cold Laser Therapy,
Acupuncture, Homeopathy, Iridology,
Osteopathy

## SWITZERLAND

**ERWIN P. LOREZ, D.C.**
135 Oberwilderstrassel
Basel, CH 4054. Switzerland
(061) 54 11 55
CHIROPRACTIC: SOT

**ARI KUCHEN, D.C.**
41, Rue De La Tour
Lausanne, CH 1004, Switzerland
(021) 20 44 65
CHIROPRACTIC: Applied Kinesiology

**211**

**CENTRE CHIROPRATIQUE**
**DRS. XAVIER & MICHELE GILLET**
**CANTOVA**
Chalet Yocamou
Grund/Gstaad, 3783, Switzerland
(30) 43 93 3
CHIROPRACTIC: Applied Kinesiology,
Acupuncture, Laser Therapy, Nutritional
Healing (vitamins), Herbs, TMJ

**CLINIQUE BON PORT/BIOTONUS**
MICHEL BARRAS
Clinique Bon Port - 21, rue de Bon Port -
CH-1820 Montreux
Chemin de Mornex 7 - CH-1007 Lausanne
21635101 or
232325
CHIROPRACTIC: Craniopathy, TMJ,
Neurological Disorganization (dislexia),
Applied Kinesiology, Sports Medicine, Foot
Reequilibration